Contexts of Midwifery Practice

Transforming Midwifery Practice links theory with practice, in the context of the skills and knowledge needed by student midwives to be fit for future healthcare delivery. Each book has been designed to help students meet the requirements of the NMC Standards of Education, Essential Skills Clusters and other relevant competencies. Each book will ensure that students learn the central importance of thinking critically about midwifery.

Series editor: Judith Jackson is a Midwifery Educator and Consultant. Previously she was Head of Midwifery Education at London South Bank University and Lead Midwife for Education for London South Bank University and Canterbury Christ Church University. She has been involved with the development and monitoring of under-graduate Midwifery curriculum in Greece.

Titles in the series:

You can find more information on each of these titles and our other learning resources at **www.sagepub.co.uk**. Many of these titles are also available in various e-book formats; please visit our website for more information.

Contexts of Midwifery Practice

Helen Muscat
Heather Passmore
Sam Chenery-Morris

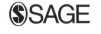

Los Angeles | London | New Delhi
Singapore | Washington DC | Boston

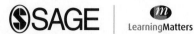

Learning Matters
An imprint of SAGE Publications Ltd
1 Oliver's Yard
55 City Road
London EC1Y 1SP

SAGE Publications Inc.
2455 Teller Road
Thousand Oaks, California 91320

SAGE Publications India Pvt Ltd
B 1/I 1 Mohan Cooperative Industrial Area
Mathura Road
New Delhi 110 044

SAGE Publications Asia-Pacific Pte Ltd
3 Church Street
#10-04 Samsung Hub
Singapore 049483

Editor: Alex Clabburn
Development editor: Richenda Milton-Daws
Production controller: Chris Marke
Project management: Swales & Willis Ltd, Exeter, Devon
Marketing manager: Tamara Navaratnam
Cover design: Wendy Scott
Typeset by: C&M Digitals (P) Ltd, Chennai, India
Printed in Great Britain by CPI Group (UK) Ltd, Croydon, CR0 4YY

Library of Congress Control Number: 2015932453

British Library Cataloguing in Publication data

A catalogue record for this book is available from the British Library

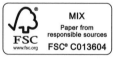

ISBN 978-1-4462-9536-6
ISBN 978-1-4462-9537-3 (pbk)

Contents

Foreword

This book is the fourth in the series on the practise of midwifery for midwifery students. As you journey through your midwifery education you will be preparing yourself to work with and care for women, their babies and families within the context of all socioeconomic circumstances. The understanding of how inequalities in health, social inclusion and exclusion impact on the health of childbearing women is an essential part of this journey.

As you read this text you will be challenged to examine your own personal belief systems so that you can truly care for all women equally. Theories of health promotion are woven throughout the book to enable you to understand the importance of individual health needs assessment to optimise health for all women.

The series addresses the requirements for midwifery education set out in the NMC Standards for Pre-registration Midwifery Education that include the Essential Skills Clusters (ESCs) and grading of practice (NMC, 2009). These Standards outline the baseline requirements of knowledge for safe and effective midwifery practice. They are designed to prepare you for contemporary midwifery practice in the UK, where midwifery care occurs in the context of a social model of care for normal childbirth. This is provided against a backdrop of government strategy and guidance (DoH, 2010; Marmot, 2010; CMACE, 2011; DoH, 2013c), statutory midwifery regulation and adherence to professional standards of practice as a midwife (NMC, 2012) and the NMC Code (NMC, 2015).

The interactive nature of this series will develop your ability to reflect and question your knowledge and practice. This will ensure that you develop professionally as a lifelong learner fully able to meet the demands of a midwifery career.

Judith Jackson, Midwifery Educator and Consultant
Series Editor: Transforming Midwifery Practice

About the authors

Sam Chenery-Morris is a senior midwifery lecturer and course leader at University Campus Suffolk. She teaches midwifery students theory in the university and supports them in practice through her link lecturer role. She examines work of other midwifery students in the UK through her external examiner role so has a thorough understanding of student midwives' needs. She has written articles for journals, presented at national and international conferences and enjoys reading and writing activities related to midwifery. Sam is the co-author (with Moira McClean) of another book in this series, *Normal Midwifery Practice*.

Helen Muscat is the Lead Midwife for Education at Canterbury Christ Church University. She is also a Supervisor of Midwives within Kent. She currently manages midwifery education within the University and has close links to the hospital Trusts that work in partnership with Canterbury Christ Church. Helen has a keen interest in public health and sociology and has been the module leader for Public Health modules within the pre-registration midwifery programmes. As a Supervisor of Midwives within Kent, Helen maintains strong links to practice and the challenges experienced by women and midwives. She has recently commenced an EdD at Canterbury Christ Church, in which she hopes to focus on women's studies.

Heather Passmore is a senior lecturer and the Lead Midwife for Education at University Campus Suffolk. With many years of experience in midwifery education, she enjoys teaching all aspects of midwifery, particularly anatomy and physiology and women's health. She is the course leader for the MA in Clinical Effectiveness and leads and contributes to a wide number of Continuing Professional Development modules. Heather has a specialist interest in reproductive sexual health which is supported by working clinically as a part-time sexual health nurse.

Acknowledgements

Sam thanks all those who have supported her in the writing of this book.

Helen thanks her husband and children for their support, and her sister Claire, and friends Karen, Jo and Bev for all the hours of inspirational discussion and debate. Not forgetting the wonderful students and women she's met and will meet in the future.

Heather thanks Sherril Hood, third year student midwife at University Campus Suffolk for sharing her work undertaken for her dissertation which included the formulation of the 'ROAD' to salutogenesis. She also thanks her husband Tim and sons Edward, Henry and James for their encouragement and tolerance during another period of academic writing.

Introduction

This new book for student midwives takes as its premise the understanding that every woman is an individual and that this individuality (of personality and preference, of age and health status and of socioeconomic circumstance) will have a profound effect on her experience of pregnancy and birth. Today's midwives provide woman-centred care in a complex world, and need to be aware of the many social, psychological and cultural influences that will impact upon that. The chapters help students explore varied and sometimes challenging situations in which midwives need to set aside their preconceptions and respond holistically to the women in their care.

Book structure

Each chapter contains a summary of the key knowledge and ideas presented, which can be used as a quick-reference guide or for revision. Suggestions for further reading and links for useful websites are given at the end.

Chapter 1 provides a context for the rest of the book by exploring salutogenesis and assessment of risk. Chapter 2 continues the emphasis on promoting health by examining how women can help to maintain an optimum BMI throughout their pregnancy and Chapter 3 looks at the care of women who are either above or below the optimum age for childbearing. Chapter 4 is concerned with aspects of communication, particularly with regard to ethnicity and difference.

Sexual health and contraception are the topics covered by Chapter 5, while Chapter 6 is concerned with mental health issues throughout the perinatal period. Chapter 7 focuses on a difficult problem, but one which the midwife may be the first professional to notice, that of domestic abuse. Chapter 8 tackles another difficult topic – that of substance misuse. Both legal substances (prescription drugs, alcohol and tobacco) and illegal drugs are considered, as is the midwife's role in educating, supporting and motivating the mother.

The final chapter, Chapter 9, looks at what happens after the birth and considers how the midwife can best use time spent with a woman during her pregnancy to help prepare and support her for parenthood.

Requirements for the NMC Standards for Pre-registration Midwifery Education

The Nursing and Midwifery Council (NMC) has established standards of competence to be met by all midwifery students in order to gain entry to the register, and these are the standards it considers necessary for safe and effective practice. In addition to the competencies, the NMC has set out specific skills that midwifery students must be able to perform at various points of an education programme. These are known as Essential Skills Clusters (ESCs). This book is structured so that it will help you to understand and meet the required competencies and ESCs. The relevant competencies and ESCs are presented at the start of each chapter so that you can clearly see which ones the chapter addresses. The boxes refer to the latest Standards for Pre-Registration Midwifery Education published in 2009 (NMC, 2009).

Learning features

Case studies and scenarios

Examples from a range of midwifery contexts, including perspectives from women and their families, have been included to help you link theory to actual practice. Some include questions to help you to think critically about how you might react in a certain situation, and to improve your decision-making skills.

Activities

There are a wide range of activities in the text to help you to make sense of, and learn about, the material being presented by the authors. Some activities ask you to *reflect* on aspects of practice, or your experience of it, or the people or situations you encounter. Other activities will help you develop key graduate skills such as your ability to *think critically* about a topic in order to challenge received wisdom, or your ability to *research a topic and find appropriate information and evidence*, and to be able to *make decisions* using that evidence in situations that are often difficult and time-pressured. Communication and working as part of a team are core to all midwifery practice, and some activities will ask you to carry out *group work activities* or think about your *communication skills* to help develop these. Finally, as a registered midwife you will be expected to *lead and manage* your own caseload or area of practice, and so some activities focus on helping you build confidence in doing this.

All the activities require you to take a break from reading the text, think through the issues presented and carry out some independent study. Where appropriate, there are sample answers presented at the end of each chapter. Remember, academic study will always require independent work; attending lectures will never be enough to be successful on your programme, and these activities will help to deepen your knowledge and understanding of the issues under scrutiny and give you practice at working on your own.

Research, theory and concept summaries

Summaries of key research, theories or concepts appear throughout the book to help you to get to grips with the evidence base in an easy-to-understand way.

Chapter 1
The principles of health promotion and salutogenesis

Sam Chenery-Morris

 NMC Standards for Pre-registration Midwifery Education

This chapter will address the following competencies:

Domain: Effective midwifery practice

Communicate effectively with women and their families throughout the pre-conception, antenatal, intrapartum and postnatal periods. Communication will include:

- listening to women and helping them to identify their feelings and anxieties about their pregnancies, the birth and the related changes to themselves and their lives;
- enabling women to think through their feelings;
- enabling women to make informed choices about their health and healthcare;
- actively encouraging women to think about their own health and the health of their babies and families, and how this can be improved;
- communicating with women throughout their pregnancy, labour and the period following birth.

Domain: Professional and ethical practice

Practise in a way which respects, promotes and supports individuals' rights, interests, preferences, beliefs and cultures. This will include:

- offering culturally sensitive family planning advice;
- ensuring that women's labour is consistent with their religious and cultural beliefs and preferences;
- the different roles and relationships in families, and reflecting different religious and cultural beliefs, preferences and experiences.

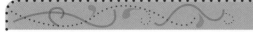

NMC Essential Skills Clusters

This chapter will address the following ESC:

Cluster: Communication

Women can trust/expect a newly registered midwife to:

3. Enable women to make choices about their care by informing women of the choices available to them and promoting evidence-based information about benefits and risks of options so that women can make a fully informed decision.

Chapter aims

After reading this chapter you will be able to:

*   understand the importance of communication in your relationship with women and their families to promote healthier lifestyles;
*   identify women in need of additional support or care;
*   consider how a salutogenic paradigm might help promote wellbeing;
*   contribute to making each contact count to promote wellbeing in the woman, baby and wider family.

Introduction

This book follows the underlying theme of the first book in this series, *Normal Midwifery Practice*, that communication between you, the midwife, and the woman is paramount. The woman and her family should be at the centre of any decisions made and you as the woman's lead professional have a duty to promote health and wellbeing for all in your care. The role of the midwife in health promotion has increased in recent years (Midwifery 2020, 2010a). This introductory chapter will focus on midwifery practice which addresses reducing inequalities in life circumstances. Life circumstances affect lifestyle behaviours. Individual attitudes, social class and economic resources, ethnicity and culture, gender and religious beliefs all affect lifestyle behaviours such as smoking, drinking, eating and breastfeeding choices to name a few.

During your midwifery education you will meet and care for women from different backgrounds to your own. The domains and Essential Skill Clusters above state that you need to promote health and wellbeing for all women and their babies respecting the different beliefs of others (NMC, 2009). Health and wellbeing are difficult terms to define as they mean different things to different people. So before we consider health promotion strategies, let's undertake an activity about your own beliefs.

What do the terms *health* and *wellbeing* mean to you? Try to discuss your answer with a friend or relative. If more than one of you is looking at the question, you are likely to have more than one answer as health and wellbeing mean different things to each of us.

Some suggested answers are given at the end of this chapter, although your answers may be very different.

Health promotion

Now you have considered some of the factors which affect health and wellbeing, such as economic, physical, emotional, spiritual and societal, you will have a better understanding of how these elements can be viewed holistically. Some people will place greater emphasis on certain aspects of their wellbeing. So you may be overweight but all the other elements of your life are positive and you consider yourself fit and well. Alternatively, if one element is missing or negative in another person's life it may affect their whole sense of wellbeing. If a woman is healthy but has poor relationships this may affect her mental health and her wellbeing. Understanding women's social, cultural and economic situations may help you to provide meaningful health promotion.

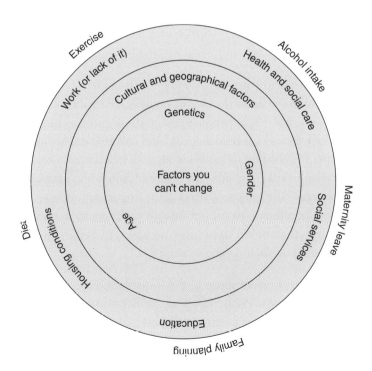

Figure 1.1: A woman's health is made up of many different elements, some of which she can make choices about while there are others over which she has little or no control

To understand how the aspects of a woman's life may be viewed holistically we will explore the terms poverty, social inclusion and exclusion and inequalities in health through a case study threaded through this chapter. Evidence will be used to show how strategies to support all women, especially those considered to be vulnerable can be implemented. The midwife does not work in isolation, therefore other disciplines and agencies and their roles in health promotion will be explored to further promote and support health. The concept of salutogenesis, which promotes wellbeing as opposed to disease, will be explored.

In the UK, around 700,000 women will give birth each year and the majority of these women will see a midwife for some or all of their care (Midwifery 2020, 2010b). In the UK the roles and responsibilities of a midwife are governed by the Nursing and Midwifery Council (NMC). Some of the most important documents that will shape your practice will come from this source, for instance: *The Midwives Rules and Standards* (2012, p15) state:

> *You must make sure the needs of the woman and her baby are the primary focus of your practice and you should work in partnership with the woman and her family, providing safe, responsive, compassionate care in an appropriate environment to facilitate her physical and emotional care throughout childbirth.*

While the Code (NMC, 2015) makes clear your personal responsibility:

> *Listen to people and respond to their preferences and concerns* (p4) and *Make sure people's physical, social and psychological needs are assessed and responded to* (p5).

Salutogenesis

One way to promote health is to consider a salutogenic framework. The term salutogenesis is made up of two words and it examines the origins (genesis) of health (salus). It was coined by a medical sociologist, who studied how people manage stress and stay healthy. As much of this chapter and indeed book focuses on reducing risk, and risk assessments which can cause stress to women, the concept of salutogenesis has been adopted by midwifery researchers and writers recently as an alternative to risk. The concept explored how some individuals stayed healthy when surrounded by stress. The effects of stress according to Antonovsky (1979) the original author, can have three manifestations on individuals: pathogenic, neutral or salutary. These three words in order mean that the effects of stress can have a bad effect, no effect or a beneficial effect on people depending on their coping strategies.

The stress experienced has to make sense to the individual, for a beneficial or salutogenic response to happen (Antonovsky, 1979). This sense, which Antonovsky calls a sense of coherence, is achieved by people who have positive reactions to the experience in one of three ways: meaningful, manageable or comprehensible. The way people cope with stress develops through their lives; some people's ability is greater than others and very much depends on their values, beliefs and the resources they have available to them, emotional, physical, spiritual and economic.

While this theory looks at major life stress, pregnancy and birth can be seen as a stress too for some women. Salutogenesis examines the underlying social, emotional and physical responses, views women holistically, to promote coping strategies and resources for better health. This theory fits with a midwifery model of care as opposed to a medical model of care. The differences between a midwifery model of care and a medical model of care can be compared to seeing birth as a normal physiological event to only normal in retrospect with the woman and midwife actively working as partners (MacKenzie Bryers and van Teijlingen, 2010). Midwives promote maternal, fetal and family wellbeing; medics look for pathology, or things going wrong. The underpinning philosophy of midwife-led care is normality, continuity of care and being cared for by a known and trusted midwife during labour (Hatem *et al.*, 2008).

Concept summary

The concept of continuity of care is sometimes used synonymously with continuity of carer. One means the same standard of care is delivered whoever gives the care. The other term means the carer is the same person who gets to know the woman and becomes trusted by her. In relation to all midwifery care, continuity of carer or case loading midwifery is the best model (Correa, 2014). Yet in most NHS Trusts continuity of care is offered instead. In relation to this book, the groups of women considered in each chapter would benefit the most from continuity of carer. As the midwife and woman build up a relationship over time, the midwife can understand the woman's life and resources and tailor individual salutogenic health promotion which best meets the woman's needs and resources.

Let us consider a case to see where the midwife can provide health promotion and how continuity of carer will help maximise the opportunities for Emma.

Activity 1.2   *Critical thinking*

Emma is 17, she smokes, has a BMI of 36, and lives with her mother and four siblings in a three bedroomed house. She is 18 weeks' pregnant when you meet her for her booking interview. She discloses her relationship with her partner and mother are turbulent and she feels down about this. She is anxious about her long-term housing as she has no personal income and the likelihood of her being re-homed despite the overcrowding in her current home is low. She tends not to go out much as she does not feel safe in her neighbourhood. As her midwife, what are Emma's challenges and how would you promote her health and wellbeing?

The answers will follow in the next paragraph as they set the scene for many of the chapters in this book.

Emma has many complex social factors. These can be viewed as potential risks for her well-being and the pregnancy or you could ask yourself, 'How can I help Emma move towards greater health?' As her midwife you will need to build up a positive trusting relationship with Emma to support her, and inform her of the best evidence for health and wellbeing. There are many challenges to this as there are a number of areas where you could and should promote a healthier diet and lifestyle for Emma. As a compassionate midwife, you also recognise reasons why Emma may not feel able to alter her lifestyle choices. Let's start by listing Emma's complex situation.

1. Her age – she should be in fulltime education.
2. She smokes – she needs information and support to reduce or stop this.
3. She is obese – she needs information about healthy eating for life and for the pregnancy duration.
4. She lives in an overcrowded house which may affect her wellbeing.
5. She is considered a 'late' booker – as she has not had pregnancy care before the 10-week gestation target, this reduces the number of antenatal appointments and opportunities to develop a good woman–midwife relationship.
6. Her personal relationships are not positive and can contribute to poor mental health.
7. She has no personal income so is reliant on the family's support.
8. She has the potential for poor mental health and social exclusion due to her relationships and unsafe neighbourhood.

Ewles and Simnett (2010) offer three models of health promotion that can be explored in relation to Emma. These are the medical model, the holistic model and wellness model (Ewles and Simnett, 2010).

The medical model

The medical approach aims to reduce mortality and morbidity by targeting high-risk groups. Emma's smoking status and obesity contribute to higher morbidity and mortality for her and her baby, thus the medical approach would aim to reduce the risks. The midwife would advise Emma of the harmful effects of smoking in pregnancy and advise her to reduce this behaviour or quit. She could refer Emma to smoking cessation services in the local area for primary prevention of diseases related to smoking. General practitioner services to support Emma to manage her weight may also be offered, along with the standard diet and nutritional advice for pregnancy offered by the midwife.

The attraction of the medical approach is that epidemiological studies have proven the association with smoking and obesity to long-term illness, so there is scientific evidence to target high-risk groups and improve their health (MacKenzie Bryers and van Teijlingen, 2010). Also, the prevention of diseases or early intervention is cheaper than the long-term treatments. This approach sees healthcare professionals as the authority or experts in health knowledge. This is problematic as it is a paternalistic view of health promotion; it focuses on disease and not health and wellbeing. It also ignores the social and environmental reasons Emma might smoke and be overweight (Sutherland *et al.*, 2013).

The holistic model

The holistic model was first introduced by the World Health Organization (WHO, 1946). It sees health as a state of physical, mental and social wellbeing, not just the absence of disease. If we use this model with Emma, physically she can be advised to adjust her diet to include five portions of fruit and vegetables a day and try to include 30 minutes of gentle exercise which would contribute to a healthier lifestyle. However, Emma's social and mental health would also be considered in this model. As Emma does not have an independent income she is dependent upon her family buying more fruit and vegetables which may be considered a luxury as opposed to an essential part of their weekly shopping. Similarly, Emma's environment, both the overcrowding at home and feeling unsafe in the neighbourhood, and poor relationships may impact upon her mental state. She may not feel able at present to alter her behaviours to improve her health; however, if she tries to eat more healthily and increase her activity level, she may improve her physical and emotional wellbeing (Claesson *et al.*, 2014). How the midwife approaches these topics might encourage Emma to change.

The wellness model

The last model, the wellness model, was introduced by the WHO again in 1984; it proposes a model of health that is a dynamic process. Here, health is the extent to which people or groups can realise aspirations and cope with change in circumstances. Social, personal and physical capabilities are reinforced. This model is related to resilience and notions of personal success in adapting to change over time. This fits with salutogenesis. The model would ask Emma how she feels about her pregnancy and what support she needs to adapt to this change in life events. She may instigate a conversation about support for change for some of her lifestyle behaviours. You may be able to support Emma in making positive life changes and there may be other professionals in your area to continue this support after her baby is born, such as the Family Nurse Partnership (FNP). The FNP works in a structured way with young women for 2 years to support their parenting, advise women about spacing their families, not having another baby soon and using the time to maximise their life changes by resuming education or skills for work.

Emma may discuss with you, her midwife, that she knows smoking in pregnancy is harmful for her baby's development and may want support to quit. Smoking cessation in pregnancy is a manageable first step for Emma, there are services to support her and she feels ready to do this. In the latest figures from the Infant Feeding Survey (2010) of the 26% of women who smoked immediately before, during or after their pregnancy, 55% gave up. The government have a target of smoking rates of 11% or less for 2015. To look at targets for health promotion and rates in your area undertake the following activity.

| **Activity 1.3** | *Research and evidence-based practice* |

Look up the Health and Social Care Information Centre online. You can look at national and local statistics on smoking cessation, smoking status at birth, healthy lifestyles, obesity and other areas pertinent to health promotion.

There are no answers at the end of this chapter as the activity is for your reference; to know where the figures are kept might be helpful for assignments or local health promotion campaigns.

The wellness model is sometimes called a client-centred approach; it is more consistent with midwifery values and salutogenesis. It places the client at the centre of the interaction. Emma would identify her own concerns and the midwife would help facilitate Emma to gain the skills and confidence to enact these. Emma may wish to stop smoking or eat more healthily and she would initiate these conversations. The midwife would support her through referrals to smoking cessation counsellors or a slimming club; the important aspect here is that Emma has decided what needs changing and not a professional. Empowerment is central to this approach (Hall, 2012). Emma will utilise her personal strength to move towards better health and wellbeing; it is not imposed on her. Empowerment is a long-term process, but Emma will develop skills that help her sustain the momentum to continue the healthier choices beyond pregnancy.

Facilitating change

Research has shown that communication styles in smoking cessation affect the success of health promotion strategies (Everett-Murphy *et al.*, 2011). In their study, three types of approaches to smoking cessation were found among the 24 nurses. The first were the 'Angry Scolders' who align to the traditional authoritarian style. If women did not comply with the health promotion the nurses scolded the women. The second approach, the 'Benign Carers', used paternalistic methods to try to persuade women to alter their behaviours, but the nurses were not convinced the women would alter their behaviour. The last approach, the 'Enthusiastic Friends', used a patient-centred approach and listened to the women's perspective. There was more interaction with the women in this group and the professionals were more optimistic of the woman's chance of success. Brief motivational interviewing was used as a strategy to enhance success.

Brief motivational interviews are used in many areas of health promotion from substance and alcohol misuse to reducing child mistreatment and weight loss (Dunn *et al.*, 2014; Thyrian *et al.*, 2010; Williams and Wright, 2014). The term brief is used as these techniques are used in a short timeframe of 5–10 minutes. Health promotion using these brief motivational interviewing skills can take place during a pre-existing appointment, such as a consultation with a GP or during an antenatal midwifery appointment. The premise of motivational interviewing is to build a rapport with individuals who wish to change their behaviours. The practitioner and client explore the effect of the undesirable behaviour. The individual client then explores how they will alter and sustain the new healthier behaviour. This approach is dependent upon the individual being at a phase in their life where they want to change and the practitioner's effective communication skills. The Family Nurse Partnership, mentioned earlier, has sustained prolonged contact with young women using motivational interviewing, rather than a brief intervention.

The Prochaska and DiClemente (1986) model of 'stages of change' is popular in understanding the stages people go through when making changes. Initially there is a precontemplation phase then four stages of change: contemplation, preparation, action and maintenance (Prochaska and DiClemente, 1986). A person is only likely to change their behaviours if they are in the contemplation phase. At the booking appointment the midwife undertakes several health promotion/screening activities. Undertake the next activity to see if you can identify these and think how you would know whether a woman is receptive to change.

Activity 1.4   *Critical thinking*

What health promotion/screening activities do you undertake at a booking appointment? Do you have the knowledge to advise women on the optimum choices and resources that might help them succeed?

Suggested answers are at the end of this chapter.

For each health promotion/screening area, the midwife is the first contact and must make this contact count. This means the midwife will offer specific health advice at that contact, even if she is referring the woman to a specialist service. It is through this communication that you will know whether the women are receptive to modifying their lifestyle behaviours. Women who are ambivalent about change are less likely to alter their behaviours. As a midwife, with a duty to promote health, asking each woman the pros and cons of each behaviour and the associated pros and cons of the change for her, is a vital step in client centred healthy promotion.

Earlier, we said Emma might initiate a conversation of her concerns and her intent to alter some of her lifestyle behaviours. However, Emma may not be aware of all the options available to her and this is where the midwife has both a health education and health promotion role. Health education is not intended to persuade women to change, but to inform them so they can make their own decisions according to their own circumstances, ability to change and values.

The educational approach provides information tailored to meet individuals' needs. To understand a woman's needs you will have made a connection with her and heard a bit about her life story. Emma's decision to cease smoking may be enhanced with knowledge if she is educated about the effects of smoking in pregnancy. Many areas of the UK use a carbon monoxide monitor to show women how much carbon monoxide (CO) they are exhaling. There are barriers and enablers to the use of CO breath tests in pregnancy (O'Connell and Duaso, 2014). Having clear referral pathways to smoking cessation services after a positive CO test is essential to support women to quit. Being sensitive and non-judgemental in your attitude to women who smoke is also essential to avoid women feeling guilty and to support them in their efforts to stop smoking.

Some midwives are concerned that the right of the woman to smoke and the trusting midwife–woman relationship is undermined by efforts to alter women's behaviours. However NICE (NICE, 2010b) says the monitoring is designed to help smoking cessation. The RCM remind midwives to care for all women in a non-judgemental way and focus on being supportive, not increasing their worry. You must also remember that increased education or knowledge does not always convert into a change in behaviour.

Social determinants

On further discussion with Emma you recognise she and her family are deprived. Her mum works in a low-paid job and the family's income is supplemented by Child Tax Credits. Most of the family are overweight and their diet does not include fruit and only limited vegetables. Emma did not succeed at her school qualifications and is worried about her future prospects. Her boyfriend works on a zero hours contract and he earns the minimum wage. Some weeks he is able to work full time, other weeks he has only 10 hours of work. He lives at home with his parents. He has limited available money to help support Emma and the baby.

Activity 1.5   *Research and evidence-based practice*

Look up the meaning of deprivation, social exclusion and poverty. See if you can find any way to measure these.

Suggested answers are at the end of the chapter.

Now we have considered deprivation and how it might be measured, let's look at how this chapter fits into the rest of the book and recent health promotion agendas. Then we will follow Emma's care through. The remaining chapters of this book each focus on a specific issue that is contemporaneous in midwifery practice. Each chapter offers an area for promoting health and wellbeing across the pregnancy and postnatal continuum as each factor/issue/topic has long-lasting effects if not identified and appropriate resources implemented in time. Each chapter is potentially connected to another in this book, as the effects of poor mental health for example may increase the chance of women misusing substances or vice versa and have a negative effect on their parenting ability. Using salutogenesis instead of focusing on risk, midwives may be able to focus on promoting health for all women. Understanding a woman's internal and external resources is essential for midwives to help women make sense of their experience and this moves the woman's sense of coherence towards wellbeing.

The reason for promoting health is to reduce maternal and fetal or neonatal mortality and morbidity. Women from socially disadvantaged groups, such as those included in this book, have poorer outcomes than more advantaged women in society (Henderson *et al.*, 2013; Lindquist *et al.*, 2013). This is not right or fair. Effective midwifery care can improve their pregnancy and life outcomes. But first let us consider the ethical principles of health promotion.

Health promotion is often used on a societal level, and can be considered paternalistic. Consider as an example childhood immunisation: if a parent decides not to have their child immunised, they are sometimes considered deviant or an irresponsible parent without understanding their reasons. There is a tension between the right of the individual to make an informed decision and the control of infectious diseases for the whole population. If midwives truly respect the women they work with, they need to understand some of these tensions through the use of ethical principles.

Ethics

Ethics is a term used to cover fundamental principles of what is right and wrong and what people should or ought to do. Ethical principles can be explored at the interactional level between midwives and women or a societal level as in what is right for a community or group. Ethics promotes good interactions between women and midwives, based on mutual respect and trust. Offering all women equitable care and promoting truly individualised information ensures each woman can make the right choice according to her needs, religious beliefs and values. Societal level ethics looks at policies and guidance such as smoking cessation, technologies such as antenatal screening and ultrasound and practices across the reproductive healthspan. The aim is to use the guidance, technology and practices to promote wellbeing, detect abnormalities or deviations from normal and improve the lives of a group of people in society. The needs of a society differ from the needs of an individual as each person will have a different set of beliefs and values and these should inform how you care for each woman. For instance while alcohol abstinence is promoted to all pregnant women, some may prefer to continue to consume alcohol despite this advice. We will look at this in a minute and in more detail in the chapter on substance misuse.

As a person you have a right to your own ethical values and beliefs. Beliefs come from various sources, our parents and upbringing, schooling, educational level and content, religious figures and the media. Most people have views on what they believe to be morally right or wrong on issues such as abortion, euthanasia or contraception. As a midwife our personal beliefs need to be set aside when offering professional midwifery care and information to pregnant women or new mothers.

Theoretically, one of the most prevalent ethical frameworks used in health care was devised by Beauchamp and Childress (2012). Their four principles were originally non-hierarchical, meaning each principle had equal weight, but now the principle of respect for autonomy is seen as paramount. This is especially relevant when midwives offer health promotion to women, as we will see.

Autonomy

The word originates from Greek to self-govern; it is often applied to midwifery practice but in ethics it means the individual is capable of deciding for themselves what matters most to them. The obligation of a midwife regarding the autonomy of a woman in her care is to respect her choices. In order for women to make informed choices the midwife shares information.

The information must be factual and complete; the midwife's role is not to bombard individual women with information but to have conversations in language they understand so they can choose which care, which tests or what health promotion message. Not giving enough information is not acceptable; it assumes you are either treating the woman as a child (paternalism) or disengaging the woman and her family actively in her care decisions. Legally information is required prior to consent, whether this is to take a blood pressure measurement, ultrasound scan or examination. If a woman lacks autonomy, her competence or capacity to consent to care may be undertaken by another person, in their best interests. This is unusual in midwifery.

Beneficence

In order to act for the benefit of others, all the available evidence must be considered. As a midwife it is your obligation to maintain contemporaneous research knowledge. As a practitioner you will know smoking in pregnancy is harmful to the woman and her developing fetus. You have a responsibility to offer smoking cessation advice (beneficence) but the woman has the right to decide whether to take this advice or not (autonomy). Her right to autonomy must be upheld, but you still have a duty to promote wellbeing. Open and honest interaction between you and the woman regarding her choices and informing her of the benefits of smoking cessation are required. The woman cannot choose to quit if she does not know the benefits of cessation for her and the baby.

Non-maleficience

Avoiding harm to others seems simple enough, yet there are many interventions in midwifery which may cause harm that should be considered. Health promotion should do no harm, but the guilt a woman experiences if she chooses not to breastfeed or declines carbon monoxide tests may be detrimental to her wellbeing. A woman may decline blood products due to her religious beliefs; the blood would do no physical harm, but her moral beliefs would be harmed in accepting it, so we need to really consider all the interventions in midwifery against the individual to know if they potentially can cause harm.

Justice

This is concerned with the distribution of healthcare, that everyone has access to a fair system. As midwives you have an obligation to treat all women equally. This means providing the same non-discriminatory care for all women, regardless of whether you agree with their decisions. Unfortunately women from lower socioeconomic backgrounds tend not to have the same access to healthcare. Sometimes they are unable to articulate their needs, or the needs of others are prioritised. You may be able to think of a time when you were torn between caring for two women, one who was able to articulate her needs and another woman. As you would not be able to meet both their needs simultaneously, one woman would have received care before the other, and it was probably the one who asked for help.

Activity 1.6   *Critical thinking*

Think about the interactions you have had with women where their values differed from your own. It may be their intention to breastfeed or not, have a water birth against medical advice, or request an elective caesarean section.

What happened when you knew about their choices, how did you feel, and how did you mask your feelings from affecting the woman's care? Having reflected, what can you do next time that may improve the interaction between you and another woman?

As this activity is based on your own experiences, there is no suggested answer at the end of this chapter. Consider though if you need to talk to your mentor, personal tutor or supervisor of midwives about any of these reflections.

Research summary

Research shows that women with decreased socioeconomic position were more likely to report that they were not treated with respect or spoken to in a way they could understand by midwives and doctors (Lindquist *et al.*, 2014). This study explored 5332 women's health seeking behaviours, pregnancy outcomes and experiences. Women who were the most deprived had less antenatal and postnatal care than more affluent women. Women in the lower socioeconomic quintile tended to be younger than 24, unemployed, of non-White ethnicity, born outside the UK, needed help to speak English, had no formal education after 16 years of age, and were single with an unplanned pregnancy.

If we follow Emma's case through, we can see she has low socioeconomic status. She is younger than 24, unemployed, with an unplanned pregnancy and has already missed some antenatal appointments. Social disadvantage is a risk factor not only for poor health in a number of ways but also for maternal death.

Research summary

Every three years the UK publishes statistics on the number of women who die in the previous three years (triennium). It also analyses reasons for these women's deaths, hence the report is published about 2 years later. The 2006–2008 UK Confidential Enquiry into Maternal Deaths shows unemployed women are six times more likely to die than employed women (Lewis, 2011). This report, showed for the first time, there has been a reduction in the inequalities

(Continued)

(Continued)

gap, with a significant decrease in maternal mortality rates among those living in the most deprived areas and those in the lowest socioeconomic group, but more must be done to keep these women safe and improve their wellbeing. The latest report from 2009–2012 included Ireland as well as the UK (Knight *et al.*, 2014); it showed maternal mortality rates are higher amongst older women, women living in the most deprived areas and women from some ethnic minority groups. There are plans to report on maternal deaths annually and for the lessons to be learned to be implemented in practice sooner. For more information on this and other work to help keep women safe look at the Mothers and Babies: Reducing Risk through Audits and Confidential Enquiries (MBRRACE) website **www.npeu.ox.ac.uk/mbrrace-uk**

The social determinants of health are the factors one has or has missing in their life that impact upon health. These include income, and status, usually afforded by employment and safe working conditions, the physical environment in which people live, their lifestyle choices and access to healthcare. If a midwife understands how these factors, particularly a lack of status, resources and poor housing affect people's health, she is better able to understand the woman's perspective. If a woman has fewer emotional and educational resources, making and sustaining a positive change can be hard. Women who have health inequalities generally have poorer health outcomes, including premature death, morbidity and their children generally have poorer health too. Many groups of women have health inequalities including women from Black and minority ethnic groups, women living in poverty, with mental health problems, those living in violent relationships, young mothers and women who misuse substances. Some women may belong to more than one of these groups; similarly just because a woman is poor does not mean she is disadvantaged and she may have a socially and emotionally fulfilling life. As the midwife, you need to understand women individually so you can tailor health promotion to their needs and not to a general idea of what any particular woman might need. This way you can really make a difference to women's lives.

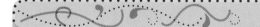

Chapter summary

This chapter introduced the concept of health promotion and health education. In order to fulfil your professional responsibility to promote healthier lives and wellbeing a salutogenic framework has been offered. This considers how women can move towards healthier lives by exploring their perception of health and making positive client-led changes. As the midwife you need to understand internal and external factors that affect the woman so she understands the situation she is in and comes to a sense of coherence about her choices. There are many areas for health promotion in midwifery practice and each woman will have individual needs. Many of the chapters in this book focus on women who are in need of additional support for inequalities in health to help them achieve their potential. This chapter is just the beginning of the approach to help women move towards their goals.

Activities: brief outline answers

Activity 1.1 Reflection [page 5]

You may have thought health means the absence of disease, such as diabetes or epilepsy. This is a common response. It may mean you eat five portions of fruit and vegetables a day, take 30 minutes of exercise five times a week, don't smoke or drink more than 14 units of alcohol per week. You may have a body mass index between 18.5–25 and consider this healthy. Alternatively you may think having friends and family, belonging to a church or other community that supports you and you enjoy being with is important to your health and wellbeing. You may have mentioned where you live, near a river or forest or within walking distance of the best nightclubs and restaurants, depending on your preferences. Having enough money to pay your bills, eat and have a little left over might also be on your list. You might have a chronic health problem, Crohn's disease or frequent migraines and still feel healthy. You might not be earning much money, as is probable during your training, but still have a sense of wellbeing.

Activity 1.4 Critical thinking [page 11]

Area for health promotion/ screening/education	Current evidence	Resources available
Smoking	Risks of smoking in pregnancy discussed with women at booking.	Smoking cessation support offered (this may be opt in or opt out).
Alcohol	Risks of alcohol consumption discussed at booking. Abstinence is the safest option.	Refer to substance misuse team if woman unable to stop drinking.
Drugs	Risks of medication from prescription drugs and illicit drugs discussed.	Refer if required to specialist services.
Domestic abuse	Screened if partner not present at booking and in pregnancy.	Referral for disclosure.
Weight	Women weighed at booking to calculate BMI.	Seen by consultant if BMI >30 or <18.
Diet	Dietary advice given regarding supplementation, foods to avoid and handling raw meat.	
Physical activity	No screening advice if woman asks about continuing aerobics class or such, otherwise not assessed.	
Mental health	Screening at antenatal and postnatal periods.	Referrals for moderate or severe illness.
Flu vaccination	Offer to all pregnant women.	

Activity 1.5 Research and evidence-based practice [page 12]

Deprivation means lack of. There are many forms of deprivation. They may include material or economic deprivation – not having any or enough financial resources. This is also called poverty. Deprivation is not the same as poverty. People can be poor but still have good positive relationships and self-esteem due to their position and roles in society.

Social deprivation is having poor or limited interactions with others. Multiple deprivations are when many areas in one's life are lacking, for example low income, unemployment, poor housing. Social exclusion is a concept associated with the above, when people are unable to be included in social and cultural activities. The reasons for exclusion are complex but can include financial, health related and access to activities.

The government measure deprivation in communities. Seven distinct domains have been identified in the English Indices of Deprivation: Income Deprivation, Employment Deprivation, Health Deprivation and Disability, Education Skills and Training Deprivation, Barriers to Housing and Services, Living Environment Deprivation, and Crime. Emma and her family score highly on many of these indices, meaning they are socially and economically disadvantaged and at risk of social exclusion or they have multiple deprivations.

Further reading

All of the below are essential documents that support your care decisions. During the course of your training it is a good idea to read these so you can provide contemporary postnatal care.

NICE (2010) *Pregnancy and Complex Social Factors.* London: NICE.

The following textbooks offer further reading on health promotion:

Dunkley, J. (2000) *Health Promotion in Midwifery.* London: Baillière Tindall.

Ewles, L. (2005) *Key Topics in Public Health, Essential Briefings on Prevention and Health Promotion.* London: Elsevier.

Useful website

www.maternal-and-early-years.org.uk/groups-with-additional-health-and-social-care-needs-during-pregnancy
Informative website from the NHS and Healthier Scotland.

Chapter 2
Weight management in pregnancy

Helen Muscat

NMC Standards for Pre-registration Midwifery Education

This chapter will address the following competencies:

Domain: Effective midwifery practice

Communicate effectively with women and their families throughout the pre-conception, antenatal, intrapartum and postnatal periods. Communication will include:

- listening to women and helping them to identify their feelings and anxieties about their pregnancies, the birth and the related changes to themselves and their lives;
- enabling women to make informed choices about their health and healthcare;
- communicating with women throughout their pregnancy, labour and the period following birth.

Refer women who would benefit from the skills and knowledge of other individuals:

- to an individual who is likely to have the requisite skills and experience to assist;
- supported by accurate, legible and complete information which contains the reasoning behind making the referral and describes the woman's needs and preferences.

Referrals might relate to:

- women's choices;
- health issues;
- social issues;
- financial issues;
- psychological issues.

Contribute to enhancing the health and social wellbeing of individuals and their communities. This will include:

- planning and offering midwifery care within the context of public health policies;
- contributing midwifery expertise and information to local health strategies;
- informing practice using the best evidence which is shown to prevent and reduce maternal and perinatal morbidity and mortality.

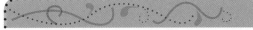

NMC Essential Skills Clusters

This chapter will address the following ESCs:

Cluster: Communication

5. Treat women with dignity and respect them as individuals.
6. Work in partnership with women in a manner that is diversity sensitive and is free from discrimination, harassment and exploitation.
7. Provide care that is delivered in a warm, sensitive and compassionate way.
8. Be confident in their own role within a multidisciplinary/multi-agency team.

Chapter aims

By the end of this chapter you will:

-   have developed your knowledge of the broad issues related to weight management during and after pregnancy;
-   understand how underweight, healthy weight, overweight and obesity are defined;
-   be aware of the midwife's role in supporting women in a person-centred way in addressing weight related issues;
-   have developed your understanding of women's concerns and anxieties about weight and body image issues.

Introduction

Quite often, when weight management in pregnancy is mentioned, the focus immediately leans towards obesity. While this is often the area of greatest concern, there are women who have difficulties with poor eating behaviours.

Maintaining a healthy weight, with appropriate gain during pregnancy, is important for both maternal and fetal health, and this chapter will explore the midwife's role in this.

Within this chapter, the care pathway related to weight management will be considered at each trimester, hopefully providing you with strategies for addressing and negotiating the issues and facilitating women in their decision-making in a positive way.

What is a healthy weight?

A healthy weight is one that lowers the risks to your wellbeing, especially the risk of:

-   stroke;
-   heart disease;

- high blood pressure;
- type 2 diabetes;
- sleep apnoea.

It is not just about the numbers achieved on weighing scales but includes lifestyles and adopting healthy attitudes and behaviours. The psychological relationship between food and weight management is well-documented. Our body image, how we view our body, is often linked to how accepted in society we feel. It impacts on our sexuality and can change and evolve throughout our life.

This said, weight is a helpful way of monitoring 'health', with the exception of mental wellbeing. The formula of the body mass index adjusts weight to height providing a more realistic overview of a person's weight. The use of this tool and others such as waist measurement should be used by healthcare professionals as part of a client-centred approach to adopting a healthy lifestyle.

To work out your BMI:
divide your weight in kilograms (kg) by your height in metres (m) then divide the answer by your height again to get your BMI
weight ÷ height = ? ÷ height =
Go to the following web page for assistance with this calculation **http://www.nhs.uk/chq/Pages/how-can-i-work-out-my-bmi. aspx?CategoryID=51&SubCategoryID=165**
If your BMI is below 18.5, you are **underweight**   If your BMI is in the range 18.5–24.9, your weight is in the **normal** range   If your BMI is in the range 25.0–29.9, you are **overweight**   If your BMI is in the range 30.0–34.9, you are **(class 1) obese**   If your BMI is in the range 35.0–39.9, you are **(class 2) obese**   If your BMI is over 40.0, you are **(class 3 or morbidly) obese**   If your BMI is over 50.0, you are **super-obese**

Figure 2.1: Body mass indicator calculation and implications

Activity 2.1   *Reflection*

Take a look around your placement area and consider whether the images used on posters are those of healthy women of different shapes and sizes. If not contact your Supervisor of Midwives and ask whether this could be discussed within the supervision forum.

As this activity is concerned with your own ideas, thought and feelings, there is no outline answer at the end of the chapter.

Body image

How women feel about their bodies is a complex issue. It is influenced by experiences during childhood, how we are valued by those around us and how we value ourselves. It is easy to blame the media and the promotion of the perfect body demonstrated through celebrity screen and sport stars. However, it is often our own values, self-esteem and level of empowerment and emotional intelligence that provide us with a perspective on the parts of our bodies that give us the most unhappiness. The media is often criticised for portraying 'ideal' women, which fosters societal acceptability of an unrealistic image. Rogers and Devon (2012) compiled a selection of stories and experiences in the name of body confidence. The resulting book *Body Gossip* aimed to encourage people to think about their bodies more, so that they might ultimately think about them less, empowering the readers to accept themselves. Chapter 4 of the book incorporates reflections from women that are both positive and negative. What is evident from their stories is that before, during, and after birth women think about their bodies and what they may look like in relation to changes in size and shape.

When you meet women for the first time they will have already established their own views and feelings about their bodies and may have considered how their changing body may make them view themselves; therefore it is vital that the topic of weight and its management is broached in a sensitive way.

Activity 2.2   *Reflection*

You can do this activity on your own, but you may find enlisting friends or colleagues will provide invaluable discussion and debate. It may provide you with the opportunity to discuss your own anxieties and thoughts about your own body image; additionally, by sharing this activity you may help to empower one another.

On a large piece of paper, create a mood board that represents how you feel about you. Choice of materials and images is entirely up to you. There is no right or wrong outcome for this activity, this is truly about 'self'.

As this activity is concerned with your own ideas, thoughts and feelings, there is no outline answer at the end of the chapter.

Women who are underweight

As a midwife, you may encounter women with eating difficulties, which may have begun in their teenage years or earlier. These difficulties can range from fussy eating habits to anorexia nervosa or bulimia nervosa. In whichever form these disorders present, the woman's mental wellbeing, relationships and fertility may have been affected. It is important to understand the enormity of the issue. The Eating Disorders website ABC (**www.anorexiabulimiacare.org.uk**) suggests that the UK has one of the highest rates of eating disorders in Europe, with 1:100 women having been clinically diagnosed with an eating disorder, which equates to 269,000 women in England and Wales. Added to this statistic are those who have issues with food, yet could not be diagnosed with a clinical condition as they did not present with significant symptomology (ABC, 2014). This support website cautiously adds that estimates vary, a conclusion which is reasonable as weight issues often remain a taboo subject for many, a factor compounded by the impact of social media on how people are expected to look and what makes them valued in society. Of more concern is the estimation that between 11–13 million people in the UK have psychological issues related to food:

- 25% of adults admit they feel guilty after eating.
- 25% of adults also say that they think they would be happier if they were thinner (when in fact they are not overweight).
- 60% women say they cannot stand the way they look.
- Only 1 in 25 is totally happy with her body.
- 1 in 6 women and 1 in 10 men regularly skip meals in an attempt to control their weight.

(ABC, 2014)

The Health and Social Care Information Centre (HSCIC, 2014b) recently announced that statistically admissions to NHS hospitals for eating disorders had risen to 2560, an increase of 8% on the previous year. However, placing this statistic in context, 9 out of 10 of these admissions were for anorexia nervosa-related conditions.

The Press has coined the term 'pregorexia', which suggests a controlling of eating during pregnancy to the detriment of the woman and unborn baby. For some eating disorders, symptoms arose in pregnancy, but for others there is a continuation of an eating disorder which is fuelled by the pregnancy. The Press suggest that it is encouraged by our fascination with celebrities and their need to be ideal in weight and body image (Mathieu, 2009). Easter *et al.* (2013) conducted a small study aimed at investigating the prevalence of eating disorders in pregnancy. They recruited a sample group of 739 women and found that 18 continued to exhibit eating disorders, with a further 37 women demonstrating eating disorders which had not been clinically diagnosed. A quarter of the sample group express their concerns about increased weight and shape changes. Although these statistics are somewhat lower than the researchers expected, it could be argued that this group of women in reality represents a much higher group, as such conditions may remain hidden from healthcare professionals and even family and friends for the fear of stigmatisation.

Activity 2.3 — *Research and critical thinking*

Consider the definition of a healthy weight and what is recommended as balanced diet and physical activity. Review NICE (2010c) Weight management before, during and after pregnancy *(NICE guideline PH27)*. National Institute for Health and Care Excellence.

continued . . .

continued . . .

Now complete the following table:

Eating disorder	Who's at risk?	Signs and symptoms	Co-morbidity
Anorexia nervosa When someone tries to keep their weight as low as possible, for example by starving themselves or exercising excessively			
Bulimia When someone tries to control their weight by binge eating and then deliberately being sick or using laxatives (medication to help empty their bowels)			
Binge eating When someone feels compelled to overeat			

You will find a completed version of this table at the end of the chapter.

NICE (2004) provides a clinical knowledge summary of eating disorders and suggests that atypical eating disorder (that is conditions other than binge eating, where a clear definition has not been possible) represent the commonest presentation followed by binge eating, bulimia nervosa and then anorexia nervosa. Overall, it is more common in women and it is estimated that they are ten times more likely to have an eating disorder than men are (Royal College of Psychiatrists, 2014).

The focus of eating disorders is the inordinate preoccupation and fear of gaining weight, body shape and size. With bulimia nervosa there is uncontrolled eating followed by compensatory purging; binge-eating disorder mirrors this without compensatory purging. Treasure (2012) highlights worrying epidemiological surveys, which show that the prevalence of women who experience some form of eating disorder in their lifetime continues to increase. The relationship between family and biological, social and cultural factors contributing to the development of eating disorders has been explored and appears to create much debate (Stice, 2002; Jacobi *et al.*, 2004; Treasure, 2012).

The cost of eating disorders to the NHS and private care was estimated at £80m–£100m in 2012. B-eat (Beating Eating Disorders, 2012) in reviewing the cost implication of eating disorders adds one caveat when considering figures, namely, that there is evidence of co-morbidities. There is a strong association with psychosis and with borderline personality disorder, and slightly less association with depression, and this increases the projected financial implications.

The diagnosis of anorexia nervosa is related to weight-to-height ratio that is less than 85% of expected weight for age and height. As with obesity, BMI is calculated, <18.5 being classed as underweight; however there is a range of thinness (e.g. from 16.0 to 18.49).

Bulimia and binge eating sufferers may have a weight within a normal range, so diagnosis will rely rather upon a combination of observing the individual's eating habits and psychological testing. Treasure (2012) calculates that a third of anorexia suffers never recover and those with bulimia or binge eating are prone to relapse.

Activity 2.4 — *Communication*

You meet Sue at her booking interview; she is 26 years old, this is her first pregnancy and you see that she has noted she had an eating disorder when she was 17.

With this information in mind, consider the conversation and the types of things you might want to discuss. Remember that she may have a normal BMI. You could start the conversation by saying, 'Some women don't like the thought of putting on weight in pregnancy – how do you feel about that?'

While you are completing this activity, consider the type of language you would use. Try to use positive words.

Nutrition	Psychological issues	Medical aspects

Some suggested answers are given in the partially completed version of this table at the end of the chapter.

Obesity

It is estimated that 25% of the adult population in the UK is obese. For many the consequences of this include diabetes, hypertension and cardiac disease. The physical issues are not the only symptoms of the growing population; obesity has implications for mental health and mental wellbeing. The complexity of being overweight or obese not only includes a physical strain, but it often impacts on one's mental health and social identity. While the causes of obesity are rudimentarily simple, that is the relationship of energy expended and taken in, the psychological relationship between human beings and food is exceptionally challenging to understand and address. Theories related to emotional eating are well-documented and at some level understood; however each person's story is often different perhaps just with similar principles. The physical consequences of obesity have a cost implication particularly to the NHS; it is estimated that by 2025 this cost will be in the region of £5 billion (Butland *et al.*, Foresight Project, 2007).

Obese women within the childbearing continuum will meet challenges relating to their weight, pregnancy and care package. There is undoubtedly a correlation between obesity and pregnancy outcome. However, it is vital that midwives focus on ensuring a positive birthing experience for all women, and care should always be person-centred rather than condition-focused. Remember that dieting in pregnancy is not recommended; therefore this should not be implied (NICE, 2010c).

A broad-brush approach to defining the care package an obese woman should have is dependent on her BMI (body mass index). Figure 2.1 showed you how to calculate BMI, and listed the differing classifications of weight/obesity according to BMI. It appears, however, that within maternity services women are classified as obese or not. The BMI calculation is the most commonly used tool to calculate body fat ratio; however, it most certainly has its limitations. BMI does not consider gender, age, and muscle mass, lean body mass or fat mass. However, it is useful as a component of the health assessment, which considers nutrition, activity, family history and body fat percentage. In midwifery practice, the usefulness and accuracy of BMI as a diagnostic tool only becomes controversial for women whose weight puts them on the borderline of certain types of admission criteria – for example those wanting to birth in a midwifery lead unit (MLU) or birth centres but whose BMI would suggest this may not be a safe option.

Waist measurement is a useful tool which works on the principle that your waist measurement should be less than half your height. It is suggested that if your abdominal fat is greater, this is more of a concern than fat which accumulates on the buttocks or breast (**Slimmersecrets.com**). Using this measurement at booking would be a useful tool as part of a holistic approach to weight management in pregnancy, but it would raise challenges as the pregnancy progresses.

Planning care with women with weight management issues throughout their pregnancy and the postnatal period

First trimester

The first trimester is the optimal time to broach the topic of weight management, as many women consider their health choices at this point of pregnancy. Micali (2007) notes that often women equate weight to self-worth, therefore while it is an optimal opportunity to discuss weight and nutrition, it is also a sensitive time as women realise there may be changes and challenges in their eating and practices.

It should be noted at this point that the venous thromboembolic risk assessment is linked to weight assessment and is a vital component of care pathway during pregnancy; however it will not be explored in depth in this chapter. NICE provide clear guidance as will your placement areas. It is very easy at a booking interview to calculate BMI and tell women what they should and shouldn't be eating. If the midwife provides a rationale for avoiding salmonella and listeria prone foods, this is merely information-giving rather than health promotion. Of course this advice should be given remembering that this broad-brush approach to health promotion may not suit all. A more holistic approach may be to discuss the food the woman normally eats, consider her budget, and how she might optimise her dietary requirements during pregnancy, explaining that these may change throughout pregnancy.

The Health Action Model

This model devised by Tones (Green and Tones, 2010) is concerned with the empower-ment of the client, and certainly lends itself to midwifery practice. It supports the midwife role in designing a holistic woman-centred package of care, which encourages women to take control over their pregnancy.

The components of this model are as follows:

Stage 1 & 2: Identify and explore the issue.
Stage 3: Help women set goals and establish the options.
Stage 4: Select an option, weigh up pros and cons.
Stage 5: Create an action plan.

Activity 2.5   *Evidence-based care and decision-making*

Consider the two women below and the advice you may offer them referring to the Health Action Model above (Green and Tones, 2010).

Jane has a BMI of 35; she is happy with her weight and her body image. She tells you that it is important to her to remain healthy throughout her pregnancy. She is also a vegetarian.

Maria has a BMI of 37; she tells you she has struggled with her weight maintenance through-out her life. She has been going to slimming club and has lost two stones prior to getting pregnant. She tells you that it is important to her not to put on too much weight in preg-nancy. She swims twice a week.

A vital part of planning care for Jane and Maria would be to have a good understanding and awareness of the services available in your area – not only within the NHS but also within the community.

Do a quick search of slimming clubs and weight management services in and outside of the health service. Then consider whether any of these are suitable for pregnant women.

Outline answers to the part of this activity that is not dependent on what is available in your own area are given at the end of the chapter.

The implications for women who are classed as obese (i.e. who have a BMI greater than 30) may vary from Trust to Trust. However, the booking interview is a prime time to introduce this topic; it is crucial that this discussion is undertaken in a sensitive way (consider the outcome of your mood board and how you feel about your body). The referral to other healthcare professionals may also apply to other groups of women such as those who have had bariatric surgery. Therefore at booking inquire whether the woman has continued to see the bariatric aftercare team. The diet of a woman who has undergone bariatric surgery will be different to those who have not; therefore it is vital that the midwife understands what this group of women will be able to eat and not eat. You will also need an understanding of the greater implications of having bariatric surgery and being pregnant. In the United Kingdom it is estimated that 8087 women choose to undergo some type of bariatric surgery (The NHS Information Centre, Lifestyles Statistics, 2012). The term bariatric surgery is an umbrella term for obesity surgery that may include gastric banding, gastroplasties, stomach stapling, gastric bypass and sleeve gastrectomy. NICE (2006a) recommends this type of surgery as suitable for those with a BMI of greater than 40 or for those with a BMI of over 35 and co-morbid health problems. In comparing surgery with non-operative management NICE (2006a) suggests surgery is more effective than a non-surgical approach. Maggard *et al.* (2008) undertook a systematic review, considering pregnancy and fertility after bariatric surgery and concluded that adverse outcomes were not as likely had they stayed obese.

Activity 2.6   *Evidence-based care and decision-making*

Take a look at the following website:

www.bospauk.org

It will give you an insight into diet and supplements that women who have undergone bariatric surgery will require.

Consider the differences between this and a normal diet.

As this activity is based on your own research, no answer is given at the end of the chapter.

With obesity figures increasing and a move towards preventative bariatric surgery performed by the NHS, it is likely that as a qualified midwife you may meet women who have undergone such surgery, therefore understanding the possible implication will enhance your practice.

Possible complications of this surgery include:

- internal hernias;
- bowel obstruction;
- band erosion or migration;
- cholelitiasis;

- hyperemesis;

- severe anaemia;

- deficiency in folates, vitamins D and B_{12};

- protein calorie malnutrition.

(Harris and Barger, 2010)

The most common of these complications are hernia and obstruction.

During the booking interview you could enquire whether the woman takes a multi-vitamin as a preventative measure to vitamin deficiencies. Consider the use of chewable vitamin C and ferrous fumate, perhaps with a liquid iron supplement. It is also recommended that 400 mcg of folic acid is taken, particularly for those who have had gastric bypass surgery. Richens and Fiennes (2010) suggest that the initial blood screening includes: serum iron/TIBC; vit B_{12}/folate; 25-OH-VitD; vit A; bone profile; urea, electrolytes and creatinine; LFTs; magnesium, zinc and copper levels. If the woman is experiencing hyperemesis, vitamin B_6 may be sensible.

It is important to discuss how the woman feels about her body changing in shape and size; while many women may have anxieties about this, for those who have undergone bariatric surgery there may be added concerns. Remember that the decision to undertake bariatric surgery may have involved much soul-searching, a decision influenced by a negative body image and poor relationship with food.

In addition to nutrition, exercise and body image the practicality of caring for women who are obese may present some challenges. Particularly for those who are obese class 3 (Figure 2.1), sensitive preparation of the woman to ensure she can meet these challenges in a well-informed way without feeling embarrassed or overwhelmed is crucial. You should take this opportunity to discuss the use of a bigger cuff to take her blood pressure, as this will ensure the accuracy of the reading. Also, talk to her about the use of transvaginal ultrasound – as ultrasound works on the premise of being as near as possible to the item being scanned, if there is a vast amount of adipose tissue, this may not be the optimal way of scanning the fetus. At booking, the midwife may identify a close family history of diabetes and this together with a raised BMI often requires a glucose tolerance test screen. Should gestational diabetes mellitus (GDM) be detected at any point, the pathway of care may alter and referral to consultant/diabetes specialist care may be necessary. It would be useful to ensure you are clear about the local guidance and parameters on these matters; if you are well-informed you can ensure the woman is too.

Current NICE (2008) guidance suggests that screening should be offered at booking to women with the following risk factors for developing GDM:

- BMI >30;

- previous macrosomic baby ≥4.5 kg or above;

- previous GDM;

- first-degree relative with diabetes;
- family origin with a high prevalence of diabetes (South Asian, Black Caribbean and Middle Eastern).

Risk factor screening is controversial – some authorities advocate universal screening for *all* pregnant women.

Reproduction in women with anorexia nervosa may be impaired during acute episodes; however many women with a history of an eating disorder eventually become pregnant. Pregnancy in women with bulimia nervosa seems to be a more common occurrence; this may be due to the symptomology of the condition, which may include a normal weight (Micali, 2008).

This is a pertinent time to reiterate that the complexities of women's views on their body image may be contextually different but remain present whether they have a condition such as anorexia or are of normal weight. For those with a past of recent eating disorder, the prospect of weight gain in pregnancy may be terrifying. It is vital that you gain an understanding that women with eating disorders have a morbid fear of fatness and that their self-worth is measured by their shape, size and appearance. Micali *et al.* (2007) undertook a large prospective cohort study in which 12,254 women were classified as to whether they had a recent or past history of an eating disorder. The researchers measured behaviours of self-induced vomiting (SIV), laxative use, exercise behaviour, thoughts and practices of dieting before and during pregnancy. For those with a recent eating disorder, they were more likely to have episodes of SIV, laxative use and over-exercising. All groups continued to experience challenging cognition regarding weight gain and body image.

Second trimester

During this trimester, the general fatigue and sickness that can occur in the first trimester usually passes. Therefore, it may be timely to revisit nutrition and exercise to re-establish good dietary habits after a few challenging weeks. You should bear in mind that appetites may increase, therefore healthy food choices should be discussed, but this should be in relation to budgetary constraints. Observing weight gain and loss in those with a history of eating disorders will provide a starting point for the conversation, without it being the focus of the whole conversation. You may like to consider at this point that the blood tests you receive from routine screening could be affected by either overeating or lack of nutrition.

Activity 2.7   *Evidence-based practice*

Design a day's meal plan which is balanced nutritionally, economically and family-focused. Include the evidence-based literature you have used to find out this information.

You could start by visiting the following NHS website: **www.nhs.uk/livewell/healthy-eating/Pages/Healthyeating.aspx**

A suggested answer to this activity is given at the end of the chapter.

You are now invited to go back to Activities 2.4 and 2.5 and to think again about Sue, Jane and Maria. Given the problems identified at booking, how might you expect their pregnancies to be progressing? Now move on to Activity 2.8 so that you can pick up their stories.

Activity 2.8 — *Critical thinking*

1. Jane is now 24 weeks' gestation, tells you she is hungry all the time and has put on 12 lb. In general she feels very well.
2. Maria is now 25 weeks and she tells you she is still going to slimming club but is using most of her food allowance on snack foods such as crisps. She is still swimming and has joined aquanatal classes. Her weight has not increased.
3. Sue is now 25 weeks' gestation and her weight has not increased at all. She tells you she is pleased that she hasn't 'fallen back into her old ways'.

What advice might you give Jane, Maria and Sue at this stage of their pregnancy?

Suggested answers to this activity are given at the end of the chapter.

Exercise during pregnancy

The advice for exercising in pregnancy should be the same for all and morbidity associated with extreme excessive exercising is concerning for the wellbeing of all women. Websites such as NHS Choices have clear practical advice. Generally, women should be advised to continue being active, with the caveat that if they have not exercised before they should not commence rigorous activity. It is also fair to say that in early pregnancy it may be challenging to continue with exercise if they experience conditions such as hyperemesis. NICE (2010c) recommend the following within their guidance dietary interventions and physical activity interventions for weight management before, during and after pregnancy. The midwife should provide the follow advice:

- Recreational exercise such as swimming or brisk walking and strength conditioning exercise is safe and beneficial.
- The aim of recreational exercise is to stay fit, rather than to reach peak fitness. If women have not exercised routinely they should begin with no more than 15 minutes of continuous exercise, three times per week, increasing gradually to daily 30-minute sessions.
- If women exercised regularly before pregnancy, they should be able to continue with no adverse effects.

During this trimester, those with a raised BMI may be offered a glucose tolerance test, which screens women for gestational diabetes mellitus (GDM). This condition is a degree of glucose intolerance during pregnancy, usually resolving shortly after delivery. During pregnancy fasting glucose levels decrease, there is an increase in fat deposition, delay in gastric emptying and increase in appetite. Additionally progressively throughout the pregnancy, postprandial glucose concentrations increase as insulin resistance increases. Normally, this is balanced by an increased production of insulin, but for some women there is an insufficient compensatory rise (Reece *et al.*, 2009).

Third trimester, planning for birth and intrapartum care

As the care pathway planned for each woman continues, the interaction with health and social care professionals generally increases. While not ignoring the issues of those who have challenges with their weight and relationship with food, they should not be treated as the condition that is, 'the obese woman' or 'the anorexic woman'. Nonetheless the risks during the birth may be increased and challenges to the simplest task such as mobility may influence the birth plan; it is therefore vital that you are able to add in elements of normality to the birth plan.

During this trimester, for all groups the birth plan should be explored, ensuring that a realistic plan is drawn together. You should be the facilitator of this, encouraging the woman to focus on what can be achieved rather than what cannot be 'allowed'. The conversation should be open and transparent, and consider the service the locality has to offer, as well as being client-centred. Should the choices made fall outside of given criteria, be open and honest that you may need to seek support and advice and come back to explore further.

For those at the lower end of the BMI scale, some of the challenges may be the issue of consuming high energy/calorie foods and drinks in labour. Therefore, this should be a key component of the discussion, exploring the rationale for doing so. A huge concern for those with body dysmorphia may be others being able to see her body naked. Therefore assure her that she will be able to wear whatever she chooses in labour, but explore what happens if an operative invention is required, mentioning the need to wear a theatre gown. This type of exploration will contribute to a positive birth experience and ensure her psychological wellbeing including the relationship she may have with her newborn.

For those who have undergone bariatric surgery, assessment of nutritional status should be drawn together. Micronutrition replacement should be revisited. In addition, it is advisable that gastric bands are loosened one or two weeks prior to delivery as a precautionary measure should general anaesthetic be required (Richens and Fiennes, 2010). Therefore, a referral to anaesthetics and bariatric services should be made. This is also an appropriate point to discuss pain, particularly non-specific abdominal pain; for this group the differential diagnosis of bowel obstruction, hernia and gastric band slippage should be taken seriously (Maggard *et al.*, 2008).

For obese women the challenges may be around monitoring in labour mobility and position in labour. Again, exploring and addressing fears and concerns will add to a positive mindset and increase birth experience satisfaction. Remember that for those who are morbidly obese activities such as a moving and handling assessment and obtaining bariatric beds and equipment may take a period of organisation, therefore planning is key.

Activity 2.9   *Reflection*

Consider the challenges during the intrapartum period and how these may be addressed. For help with this activity review Chapter 7 by Rajasingam and Swamy in Richens, Y. and Lavender, T. (eds) (2010) *Care for Pregnant Women Who Are Obese*. London: Quay Books.

Reflect on what you would discuss with the woman and what midwifery practice knowledge is. Identify areas of your own practice that have been enhanced by this knowledge.

As the answers to this activity depend on your own responses, there is no outline answer at the end of the chapter.

Postnatal period onwards

The impact of birth on women's bodies varies. Some will have no stretch marks, minimal weight gain, and little birth trauma to the vagina, perineum or abdomen. Others have a mixture or all of these changes to their body. For the woman who has a poor relationship with her body, these changes can lead to high anxiety and responses that include under- or over-eating. It is not possible to predict which women will respond in which way, and in fact, any women could react in a negative way to such changes. It is fair to suggest there is a high level of probability that the women who already face challenges related to weight gain or eating disorders are more likely to respond in a negative way. Orbach and Rubin (2014) raise concerns about the intergenerational transmission of body and eating problems and suggest that there is an opportunity during this period to address the issues and challenges, promoting optimal attaching and bonding between the mother and baby, ensuring the mother is not preoccupied with insecurities and anxieties.

During this period, there is a level of interprofessional collaboration required. Some women may be seen for only 10 days after the birth, therefore collaboration with the health visitor is a priority. The GP is well-placed at the 6–8 week check-up to continue or initiate interventions that promote healthy eating and exercising behaviours.

As a midwife, you should discuss the way forward concerning diet and exercise, creating a plan that takes into consideration physical recovery from the birth, time adapting to motherhood and addressing body issues such as obesity. Knowing the local resources would be helpful; some GPs might facilitate weight management programmes or provide access to health clubs. Slimming clubs may have programmes for lactating women.

For those who have previously had bariatric surgery, dietary advice may need to be reviewed, and referral may be made for interventions such as refilling of gastric bands. For those in the super-obese category (BMI >50) a more rigorous programme of intervention of weight management should be encouraged. Honest and open discussion about mortality and morbidity is vital. Marshall *et al.* (2012) found that in comparison to those who are regarded as morbidly obese or obese, the super-obese are at significant increased risk of perinatal complications. There is a cascade of risk that begins in pregnancy with increased risk of pre-eclampsia, diabetes and fetal macrosomia, developing onwards to instrumental delivery or caesarean section where there is an increased risk associated with regional and general anaesthetics. In the postnatal period, there is a higher risk of deep vein thrombosis and wound infection due to depleted skin integrity, all of which impacts on the newborn and the family.

You are now invited to go back to your previous work on planning care for Jane, Maria and Sue. What do you need to bear in mind for the postnatal period?

Activity 2.10   *Critical thinking*

Consider the information you have already gained about Jane, Maria and Sue. In the context of what you already know, how would you plan care for them now:

1. Jane has now had her baby. She gained 20 lb during her pregnancy. You visit her when she is 10 days postnatal, and she says she is concerned about losing this weight.
2. Maria had her baby by caesarean section 12 days ago. Although she only put on 12 lb during the pregnancy, she is concerned about not being able to undertake physical activity.
3. Sue had a normal delivery 6 days ago and is pleased she fits into her size 10 jeans. She also tells you she is walking at least 2 miles a day and has bought a pram that is designed to run with.

Suggested answers to this activity are given at the end of the chapter.

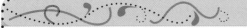

Chapter summary

This chapter has introduced the concept of healthy weight and some of the controversies related to how we measure this have been discussed. The main types of eating disorder women may experience before, during and after pregnancy have been explored and the considerations that arise in relation to the woman's wellbeing. No specific pathway has been suggested for this group of women, as the decision should be made in partnership with women utilising your own local guidance. You have been encouraged to explore your own feelings about your own body image, which on reflection should help you to understand the need to approach weight-related issues sensitively. This should be done with an appreciation of the anxieties and vulnerability such issues can raise for women without detracting from caring for their health and wellbeing.

Activities: brief outline answers

Activity 2.3 Research and critical thinking [page 23]

Eating disorder	Who's at risk?	Signs and symptoms	Co-morbidity
Anorexia nervosa When someone tries to keep their weight as low as possible, for example by starving themselves or exercising excessively	Females Teenagers Those who have experienced sexual/domestic abuse Family history High level sports person	Dieting despite being thin Obsession with calories, etc. Pretending to eat or lying about eating Preoccupation with food Food rituals Dramatic weight loss Feeling fat, despite being underweight Fixation on body image Using diet pills, laxatives or diuretics Vomiting/purging Excessive exercising	Severe mood swings Dizziness, fainting and headaches Growth of fine hair all over the body and face Depression Dry, yellowish skin and brittle nails Slowed thinking; poor memory Constipation Tooth decay and gum damage Lack of energy and weakness Organ failure and death
Bulimia When someone tries to control their weight by binge eating and then deliberately being sick or using laxatives (medication to help empty their bowels)	Those who have problems with anxiety, depression and impulse control	No control over eating Eating large amounts with no change in weight Secret eating Stashes of food hidden Alternating between overeating and fasting – all or nothing approach	Weight gain Abdominal pain and bloating Chronic sore throat Broken veins in eyes and face from vomiting Weakness and dizziness Ruptured stomach or oesophagus Acid reflux or ulcers Tooth decay and mouth sores Swollen cheeks and salivary glands
Binge eating When someone feels compelled to overeat	Poor psychological relationship with food, often triggered by a stressful event	No control over eating Eating large amounts with no change in weight Secret eating Feeling of disgust and self-loathing	Type 2 diabetes Gallbladder disease High cholesterol High blood pressure Heart disease Certain types of cancer Osteoarthritis Joint and muscle pain Gastrointestinal problems Sleep apnoea

Activity 2.4 Communication [page 25]

The suggestions given here for how you might talk to Sue do not represent an exhaustive list, so continue to add more.

Nutrition	Psychological issues	Medical aspects
What's your favourite snack/dinner/treat?	Some people can't eat when they feel stressed/sad/ill; do you?	I see you've written down you had an eating disorder in your first pregnancy; I would be interested to know about your experiences?
When you go out for a meal what type of food do you go for?	Has anyone told you how lovely you look now you are ** weeks' pregnant? Do you think you look good?	
I see you've written down you had an eating disorder in your first pregnancy; how is it this time round? *This encourages their thoughts about the situation.*	I see you've written down you had an eating disorder in your first pregnancy; do you think it will be the same this time? *This focuses on their thoughts not yours.*	I've noticed that you have a large amount of ketones in your urine; this worries me, would it be ok to talk about why this might be? *This allows the person the opportunity to say no*
In this leaflet about diet, is there anything you will miss eating?		

Activity 2.5 Evidence-based practice and decision-making [page 27]

Using the stages of Green and Tones's Health Action Model:

Jane

Stage 1 & 2: Jane's BMI places her in the obese class 2 category, therefore this may impact on options available to her such as attending a midwifery lead unit or a waterbirth. Discuss how important this may be to her. She may also need a more in-depth blood screen; again would she mind this? Does she already take any supplements?

Stage 3: Discuss ways that this can be addressed within your area of practice and who might help you both do this – Supervisor of Midwives, Consultant Midwife or Specialist Midwife. Regarding blood screen, do you need to talk to someone in the path lab?

Stage 4: Chat through pros and cons.

Stage 5: Document the discussion and plan if any.

Maria

Stage 1 & 2: Maria's BMI places her in the obese class 2 category, therefore this may impact on options available to her such as attending a midwifery lead unit or a waterbirth. Discuss how important this may be to her. Discuss whether she is still attending a slimming club; if not, does she want to? Does she want to join any pregnancy-specific water type exercise classes?

Stage 3: Discuss ways that this can be addressed within your area of practice and who might help you both do this – Supervisor of Midwives, Consultant Midwife or Specialist Midwife. Do you or any of your team members or GPs have contacts with slimming clubs or aquanatal class teachers?

Stage 4: Chat through pros and cons.

Stage 5: Document the discussion and plan if any.

Activity 2.7 Evidence-based practice [page 30]

You could start by visiting the following NHS website: **www.nhs.uk/livewell/healthy-eating/Pages/Healthyeating.aspx**, and consider the use of the Eatwell plate.

Activity 2.8 Critical thinking [page 31]

Jane

- Share your knowledge of healthy snacking choices.
- Would she like a dietitian referral?
- Is there a type of exercise she used to enjoy which she might like to do now? If so does she have any questions of concerns about doing this?
- Consider the local guidance in relation to serial scan criteria.

Maria

- Consider how you can give her positive reinforcement for her achievement.
- Inquire about how much exercise she is actually doing to ensure she is not over-exercising.
- Discuss fluid intake to ensure she remains well hydrated before, during and after exercise.

Sue

- Again consider how you can give her positive reinforcement, as this issue is obviously really important to her.
- You could ask her how she has achieved this, which may lead into a discussion about her diet and exercise regime. From this you can decide whether there are any dietary or exercise concerns.
- Take advice about her BMI being so near the lower end of the 'normal' range at booking, which at 25 weeks may mean she has lost a little bit of weight.

Activity 2.10 Critical thinking [page 34]

Again the priority here is how you share your concerns; it should be in a constructive way so as to encourage positive attitude and actions.

So for Jane perhaps consider the following:

1. Discuss her expectations of weight loss and try to add perspective to her ideas by encouraging a 1–2 lb loss per week.
2. As she is a vegetarian she might need to reassess the content of her diet. Perhaps discuss websites which offer a balanced diet approach.
3. Encourage exercising in a gentle way to start; perhaps you know the contact for mother and baby groups which offer yoga or something similar.

For **Maria:**

1. It might be useful to discuss her caesarean section to ensure she understands the body's response to surgery.
2. It might be helpful to plan a gentle regime of exercise once she is well enough to begin exercising.
3. She might benefit from linking her GP/health visitor into this plan, seeking support and further guidance, particularly if she wishes to return/continue attending the slimming club.
4. Chatting through the benefits of a healthy diet and fluid intake would bring the conversation together.

For **Sue:**

1. It may be useful to refer to Sue's previous conversation, where she referred to falling into her old ways. You could use this as a point of reference to enquire if she feels she may be losing control of her previous healthy eating and exercising plans.

2. She may find it useful to discuss this with the GP/health visitor.
3. The aim of the conversation is to aid Sue with assessing the situation and gaining perspective on the situation.

Of course, should you feel in any of the cases above there are issues that are creating grave health concerns, you should discuss with the GP and health visitor. Conversations would be documented too.

Further reading

Easter, A., Bye, A., Taborelli, E., Corfield, F., Schmidt, U., Treasure, J. and Micali, N. (2013) Recognising the symptoms: how common are eating disorders in pregnancy? *European Eating Disorders Review*, 21: 340–344. doi: 10.1002/erv.2229.
A useful article which can inform your practice.

Green, J. and Tones, K. (2010) *Health Promotion: Planning and Strategies*. London: SAGE.
This book will provide a well-rounded exploration of health promotion and encourage you to think outside the box, valuing one size does not fit all.

Harris, A.A. and Barger, M.K. (2010) Specialized care for women pregnant after bariatric surgery. *Journal of Midwifery & Women's Health*, 55 (6): 529–539.

NICE (2004) Eating disorders: core interventions in the treatment and management of anorexia nervosa, bulimia nervosa and related eating disorders (NICE guideline CG9). National Institute for Health and Care Excellence.

NICE (2010) Weight management before, during and after pregnancy (NICE guideline PH27). National Institute for Health and Care Excellence.

Richens, Y. and Lavender, T. (eds) (2010) *Care for Pregnant Women Who Are Obese*. London: Quay Books.
See especially Chapter 7 by Rajasingham, D. and Swamy, S. 'Intrapartum care of obese women'.

Rogers, R. and Deven, N. (2012) *Body Gossip*. Rickshaw Publishing.
This book is an easy read which provides the views of real women.

Useful websites

www.anorexiabulimiacare.org.uk
Anorexia and bulimia care.

www.bospauk.org
British Obesity Surgery Patient Association (2014).

www.nhs.uk/livewell/healthy-eating/Pages/Healthyeating.aspx
NHS Choices: healthy eating.

www.rcpsych.ac.uk/healthadvice/problemsdisorders/eatingdisorderskeyfacts.aspx
Royal College of Psychiatrists (2014).

Chapter 3
Age and childbearing

Heather Passmore

 NMC Standards for Pre-Registration Midwifery Education

This chapter will address the following competencies:

Domain: Effective midwifery practice

Communicate effectively with women and their families throughout the pre-conception, antenatal, intrapartum and postnatal periods. Communication will include:

- listening to women and helping them to identify their feelings and anxieties about their pregnancies, the birth and the related changes to themselves and their lives;
- enabling women to make informed choices about their health and healthcare;
- actively encouraging women to think about their own health and the health of their babies and families, and how this can be improved.

Determine and provide programmes of care and support for women which:

- are appropriate to the needs, contexts, culture and choices of women, babies and their families;
- are made in partnership with women;
- involve other healthcare professionals when this will improve health outcomes.

Domain: Developing the individual midwife and others

Demonstrate effective working across professional boundaries and develop professional networks by:

- effective collaboration and communication;
- sharing skills.

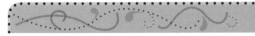 **NMC Essential Skills Clusters**

This chapter will address the following ESCs:

Cluster: Communication

Women can trust/expect a newly registered midwife to:

1. Be attentive and share information that is clear, accurate and meaningful at a level which women, their partners and family can understand:

continued . . .

continued . . .

- articulates a clear plan of care, that has been developed in partnership with the woman;
- communicates effectively and sensitively in different settings, using a range of methods and styles in individual and group settings.

3. Enable women to make choices about their care by informing women of the choices available to them and providing evidence-based information about benefits and risks of options so that women can make a fully informed decision:

- uses appropriate strategies to encourage and promote choice for all women;
- provides accurate, truthful and balanced information that is presented in such a way as to make it easily understood;
- respects women's autonomy when making a decision, even where a particular choice my result in harm to themselves or their unborn child, unless a court of law orders to the contrary;
- discusses with women local/national information to assist with making choices, including local and national voluntary agencies and websites.

8. **Be confident in their own role within a multidisciplinary/multi-agency team:**

- consults and explores solutions and ideas appropriately with others to enhance care;
- works inter-professionally as a means of achieving optimum outcomes for women.

Chapter aims

After reading this chapter you will be able to:

- explain the demographic patterns of age and childbearing;
- promote a salutogenic approach to pregnancy and childbearing for women at either end of the age spectrum for childbearing;
- discuss the factors influencing conception at either end of the age spectrum;
- detail the needs and difficulties of childbearing at either end of the age spectrum;
- review action and support that a midwife may provide, with other agencies, to promote normality in childbearing to these women and their families.

Introduction

Government statistics report the age range for childbearing as 15–44 years (ONS, 2014), reflecting a time between menarche and the menopause with some correlation to average age of first intercourse and the onset of peri-menopausal symptoms in women. While the average age of menarche is declining, it is currently 12.7 among Caucasian girls and 51 is the average age for the menopause (Jones *et al.*, 2014). The optimum time for women to have children is between the ages of 20 and 35 (RCOG, 2009b), therefore women conceiving while a teenager, particularly under the age of 16, and those over 35 are regarded by obstetricians to be at higher risk of complications. In the years between 1990 and 2010 concern has been directed at the high teenage pregnancy rate in the UK; however as these rates are now declining attention is directed to the increasing age of women giving birth and associated awareness to declining fertility beyond the age of 35. This chapter will explore the experiences and challenges of pregnancy and childbearing at either end of the childbearing age spectrum. It will provide midwives with the information needed to promote a healthy pregnancy.

In the 1990s the United Kingdom was recognised as the European country with the highest teenage pregnancy rate, nine times that of the Netherlands and half that of the United States of America (SEU, 1999). This gave rise to detailed study of and interventions of a multi-agency nature, that would effect a reduction in this rate. Over a ten-year period from 2000, the UK government proposed a 50% reduction in teenage conceptions. Although this rate has not been achieved, significant success has been made with a 41% reduction in conceptions in under 18-year-olds since 1998 (ONS, 2014). Teenagers who do conceive, however, are at risk of poor child health outcomes, poor maternal emotional health and wellbeing, and an increased risk of living in poverty (DCSF, 2010).

By contrast the average age of women giving birth in the UK has been increasing for the last three decades (see Figure 3.1), now reaching 30 years old (ONS, 2014). This trend is replicated throughout high resource countries worldwide (Cooke *et al.*, 2011). Over 50% of babies born in England and Wales in 2014 were born to mothers over 30 years old.

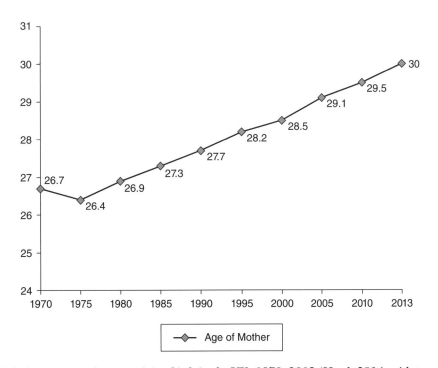

Figure 3.1: Average age of women giving birth in the UK, 1970–2013 (Hood, 2014, with permission)

Activity 3.1   *Research and evidence-based practice*

Go to the link **www.ons.gov.uk/ons/dcp171778_353922.pdf** and retrieve the document *Conceptions in England and Wales, 2012.*

Look at Figure 1 on page 3 of the above document. This shows a considerable increase in the conception rate for women aged 35 years and over, which is even more marked in women over 40.

Look at Figure 2 on page 5. This graph shows the changing rates in pregnancy for women aged under 18 and over 39, taking the date of 1990 as a base of 100%.

What explanations can you propose for these changes?

Look at Figure 3 in the same document. What does this tell you about the conception rate in women under 18 years old?

As the answers to this activity inform the discussion that follows, they will be included in the text below.

While the overall birthrate showed a decline of 2.7% between 2011 and 2012, the under-18 conception rate for 2012 is the lowest since 1969; however 49% of all conceptions to women aged under 18 led to an abortion. The conception rate for women aged 35 years and over has increased by 90% while that of women aged 40 and over has more than doubled since 1990, from 6.6 to 14.0 conceptions per thousand women. Conceptions leading to abortion in these age groups fell from 43% in 1990 to 28% in 2012 (ONS, 2014). Over the last two decades the percentage of conceptions leading to a legal abortion has generally increased for women aged under 20, but decreased for women aged 35 and over. There is no evidence to suggest that women use abortion as a method of contraception and for some women it can cause lasting impact on their wellbeing (Hoggart and Phillips, 2010; National Collaborating Centre for Mental Health, 2011).

While the average age of women giving birth is increasing there is a marked decrease in the teenage pregnancy rate (ONS, 2014: Figure 3). The size of the female population of childbearing age (women aged 15–44) influences the number of conceptions. The composition of the female population will also influence the number of conceptions as there are peak age groups for giving birth (25–29 and 30–34), and abortions are most prevalent between 20–24 years of age. The relative size of these groups will impact upon the number of conceptions. Changes in the size of the population are determined by births of females in previous years, mortality and migration.

Factors which can explain the reduction in teenage conceptions include:

- Investment by successive governments to improve and make sex and relationships education a legal requirement, improved access to contraceptives and better publicity about contraceptive and sexual health services.

- A shift in aspirations of young women towards education (Broecke and Hamed, 2008). Getting more teenage parents into education, training or employment, to reduce their risk of long-term social exclusion was a major goal of the Social Exclusion Unit report (SEU, 1999).

- The perception of stigma associated with being a teenage mother (McDermott *et al.*, 2004). Gingerbread, a national organisation for single parents, irrespective of their age, have identified many judgemental comments expressed about single parenting (Gingerbread, 2014; BBC, 2014).

Teenage pregnancy can be seen as a cause of health inequalities and child poverty. A comparison of rates across regions in England shows that the North East had the highest under-18 conception rate in 2012 while the South East and the East both had the lowest rate with 23.2 per thousand women (ONS, 2014).

Factors that can affect age at childbirth

Teenage pregnancy

Is associated with:

- poverty;
- being in the care system (Looked After Child);
- having a teenage mother;
- low educational achievement;
- poor employment prospects;
- mental health problems;
- involved in crime;
- Black or ethnic minorities;
- suffered/suffering abuse;
- low self-esteem.

(SEU, 1999)

Pregnancy at advanced maternal age

Is associated with:

- increased participation in higher education;
- increased female participation and aspiration in employment;
- the increasing importance of a career;
- the rising opportunity costs of childbearing;
- waiting for greater financial security;
- labour market uncertainty;
- housing factors;
- instability of partnerships/not yet met the right partner.

(Jefferies, 2008; Ní Bhrolcháin, 2012)

Significant efforts and resources have been invested to reduce the teenage pregnancy rate. While pregnancy and childbirth for older women may also present particular challenges, with some mothers requiring additional support, it can be questioned whether society should provide the services that they need, rather than attempt to cajole women into having children earlier than they feel is right for them.

Effect of age on pregnancy, birth and parenthood

Teenage mothers

The teenage mother is more likely to be a lone parent, suffer a postnatal depression rate three times higher than that of older mothers, with a risk of poor mental health for three years after the birth. The child of a teenage parent has a 60% higher rate of infant mortality than that of babies born to older mothers, is more likely to be of low educational attainment, live in poor housing and experience poor health and have lower rates of economic activity in adult life. However, 20% of births conceived to under-18s are to young women who are already teenage mothers (DCSF, 2007).

It is widely understood that teenage pregnancy and early motherhood can be associated with poor educational achievement, poor physical and mental health, social isolation, poverty and related factors. There is also a growing recognition that socioeconomic disadvantage can be both a cause and a consequence of teenage motherhood (Swann *et al.*, 2003).

In 2000, the UK government set a target to halve the teenage conception rate by 2010, when compared with 1998. Local authorities set ten-year strategies in place, aiming to reduce the local rate between 40% and 60%. These local targets were to help underpin the national 50% reduction

Physical	Psychosocial
Anaemia	Late booking for antenatal care
Pre-eclampsia and eclampsia	Teenage mothers are the most likely of all age groups to smoke (see Chapter 8 for effects of smoking on pregnancy)
Pregnancy induced hypertension	
Prolonged and difficult labour	Missed opportunity for pre-conception and early pregnancy health advice such as folic acid/vitamin D supplementation, dietary advice
Increased risk of spontaneous abortions in subsequent pregnancies	
	Concealed pregnancy

Table 3.1: Complications of teenage pregnancy

target. The Teenage Pregnancy Strategy ended in 2010; however teenage pregnancy has remained an area of policy interest. The current Conservative Government has included the under-18 teenage conception rate as one of its three sexual health indicators in its Public Health Outcomes Framework (2013–2016) and it is one of the national measures of progress on child poverty. This ensures a continued focus on preventing teenage conceptions as well as the social impact upon teenage mothers.

More recently Gupta (2008) has identified that the risk to primiparous teenagers is low, except for the risk of preterm birth for very young teenagers. Stapleton (2010) suggests that teenage pregnancy may confer health benefits such as protection against breast cancer and diabetes and when pregnancy is straightforward experience less obstetric intervention than older women. Many of the bullet points of pregnancy complications for teenagers are arguably no more serious than many of the risks faced at the other end of the childbearing spectrum. Biologically, there is no reason why a teenage pregnancy should not have a good outcome if pregnancy is well-managed. The problem is that because of their circumstances, teenage mothers tend not to have well-managed pregnancies; they may face huge problems of family conflict, likely change of care or fostering arrangements, relationship stress or breakdown, and problems with education, housing and money. For some teenagers this can lead to a concealed pregnancy, the young woman presenting in accident and emergency services with abdominal pain or giving birth unattended, possibly in unsuitable circumstances such as a toilet. In this situation no antenatal care will have been received so emergency care will be needed to ensure the wellbeing of mother and baby and make arrangements for postnatal care. Once a teenager has accessed care, even if she books late, the midwife can promote a salutogenic road to parenthood (see Figures 3.2 and 3.3 below).

Complications of pregnancy at advanced maternal age

Reasons for women conceiving at an older age are thought to include later marriage, and increased higher education and employment opportunities, allowing women to achieve stability and independence before deciding to have children (Page, 2011). Other factors may include reduced fertility (te Velde and Pearson, 2002), resulting in only managing to conceive at a later age, and possibly with the help of assisted reproductive technology, which can increase the likelihood of multiple pregnancies for these women (Biro *et al.*, 2012), dependent on current in vitro fertilisation (IVF) policy. The National Institute for Health and Care Excellence (NICE) amended their guidelines in 2013 to increase the upper age at which they recommend IVF treatment should be offered to 42 (NICE, 2013a). This decision was taken due to several factors; many women naturally conceive between the ages of 40 and 42, and the success rates of IVF in the last decade has meant that cost-effective treatment can now be offered. However in other countries no such age limit exists, resulting (in the rare event) of a woman giving birth in her 60s.

Current IVF policies favour the implantation of one good blastocyst under the age of 40, and two embryos being transferred in women over 40, though the risks of multiple pregnancy must be explained to the woman and her partner (NICE, 2013a).

However, choosing to delay childbirth can unintentionally have other consequences; after the age of 35 women are at increased risk of complications, interventions and adverse outcomes (Yangmei, 2014). This is generally why advanced maternal age is defined as 35 years old and over.

Some of the complications seen by women of advanced maternal age are due to existing health problems, such as hypertension and diabetes (Ecker, 2014). However, childbearing at an older age can also put women at greater risk of pregnancy induced hypertension (Carolan, 2013) and gestational diabetes (Biro *et al.*, 2012; Cleary-Goldman *et al.*, 2005).

One of the most widely known risks for women of advanced maternal age is the increased chance of conceiving a baby with Down's syndrome, or other genetic abnormalities (Forrester and Merz, 2003; Hollier *et al.*, 2000), which consequently increases the number of older women who undergo antenatal fetal testing such as amniocentesis or chorionic villus sampling; tests which are known to have miscarriage rates of one to two percent (NHS Choices, 2013b).

Other pregnancy complications and adverse outcomes associated with advanced maternal age include placenta praevia (Biro *et al.*, 2012; Cleary-Goldman *et al.*, 2005), placental abruption (Cleary-Goldman *et al.*, 2005), pre-eclampsia (Delbaere *et al.*, 2007), preterm birth (Delbaere *et al.*, 2007; Edge and Laros, 1993) and post-term birth (Roos *et al.*, 2010), low birth weight (Hoffman *et al.*, 2007; Gilbert *et al.*, 1999), stillbirth (Bateman and Simpson, 2006; Nybo Andersen *et al.*, 2000), post-partum haemorrhage (Edge and Laros, 1993), and severe maternal morbidity (Knight *et al.*, 2014). Breech presentation (Jolly *et al.*, 2000) and caesarean section (Treacy *et al.*, 2006; Cleary-Goldman *et al.*, 2005; Gilbert *et al.*, 1999) are also increased prospects for women of advanced maternal age.

As well as adverse consequences to delayed childbearing, research has also shown that there are specific advantages to having children at a later age, when women may be more emotionally mature, have better parenting skills, and be financially secure (Bornstein *et al.*, 2006; Byrom, 2004; Stein and Susser, 2000). A longitudinal study carried out in the UK between 2001 and 2007, which observed over 78,000 children, found that increasing maternal age was associated with improved health and development for children up to 5 years of age (Sutcliffe *et al.*, 2012). In particular these children had fewer accidental injuries and fewer social and emotional problems across the complete social spectrum.

There is currently a prospective randomised controlled trial in progress, which is studying the effect of a policy of induction of labour at 39 weeks' gestation for nulliparous women over the age of 35 at expected date of delivery (Nottingham Clinical Trials Unit, 2013). This trial will examine whether perinatal outcomes are improved, and whether the caesarean section rate is affected. This type of research is looking to make pregnancy and childbirth safer for older women in the future.

Teenagers and women of advanced maternal age are groups who are generally treated as 'high risk' cases and maternity care is consultant led due to the increased risks reported by the various research studies carried out (RCOG, 2009b). The NICE antenatal clinical guideline 62 (NICE, 2010a) recognises that teenagers and women aged over 40 years usually require additional care to the basic care detailed in the guideline. This approach is one that these women do not always understand, as they are often in good physical health with their only risk factor being their age and Hunter (2013) challenges the risk/negative discourse of the last 15 years in relation to teenage pregnancy.

Activity 3.2   *Critical thinking*

Access the article by Louise Hunter on the discourses of teenage motherhood, parts 1 and 2 published in *Essentially MIDIRS* in March and April 2013.

Hunter, L. (2013) Discourses of teenage motherhood: finding a framework that enables provision of appropriate support.

Part 1: Risk discourses and the shortcomings of the Teenage Pregnancy Strategy. *Essentially MIDIRS*, 4 (3): 32–37.

Part 2: Situational and developmental perspectives. *Essentially MIDIRS*, 4 (4): 32–37.

Consider how Hunter challenges the dominant ideology surrounding teenage pregnancy and how this may distort the reality of teenage motherhood. Does this fit with your experience of young mothers – have you seen young mothers choosing to become pregnant, having positive healthy pregnancies and becoming good mothers?

Discussion point: Could you envisage that as the teenage pregnancy rate falls and the average age of birth increases, there will be a shift towards a negative discourse of older age childbirth despite some recorded benefits in parenting skills? What would be possible explanations for this?

As this activity is based on your own research, no answer is given at the end of the chapter.

Salutogenesis and women at either end of the age span: the midwife's role

Salutogenesis is the theory of movement towards health and the relationship between health, stress and coping (Antonovsky, 1979). The pregnant teenager or woman of advanced maternal age begins her pregnancy journey surrounded by risks regardless of her physical health, and has to work towards, or prove to herself and others, her wellbeing. Salutogenesis when applied to midwifery proposes that midwives are in a privileged position with the responsibility to build women's confidence and self-esteem, and the knowledge to provide health promotion and influence their expectations for optimal birth (Sinclair and Stockdale, 2011). The context of care for women at either end of the childbearing spectrum requires the midwife to use the theory of salutogenesis to guide and support along the road to wellbeing and normalisation.

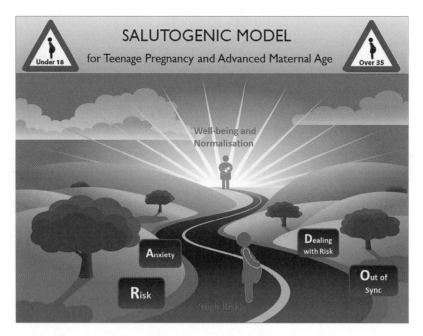

Figure 3.2: Towards a salutogenic model of care for teenage pregnancy and women of advanced maternal age (reproduced from Hood, 2014, with permission)

The significance of the 'road' and signs is to detail the journey that women at either end of the age spectrum may take during childbearing. The red triangular warning signs signify the view of obstetricians to their pregnancies. The challenge for midwives and obstetricians is to respond to the concerns of these different age groups to provide information, advice, care and support that promotes wellbeing and the normalisation of pregnancy, thus changing the triangular warning sign to a rectangular blue information sign. The four 'ROAD' themes: Risk, Out of Sync, Anxiety and Dealing with Risk that were identified for women of advanced maternal age providing risks to pregnancy and parenthood (Hood, 2014) also had relevance to teenage women and points relevant to each of these themes are identified for each end of the age spectrum in Table 3.2.

Themes	Teenage mothers	Women of advanced maternal age
Risk	Biologically immature, small pelvis, possible incomplete invasion into endometrium of chorionic villi resulting in hypertension; adverse maternal and fetal outcomes	Biologically aging ovum, leading to increased risks of congenital abnormality; declining fertility/infertility; adverse maternal and fetal outcomes
Out of sync	Societal perception; social isolation; lack of finance to support self and new family; education delay	Societal perception; loneliness, lack of social support; embarrassed being an older mother; friends and family had children earlier

Anxiety	Ability to cope as a mother, impact on education, housing – rejection from family home or current social care; finance	Coping with the physical demands of motherhood; previous pregnancy experience, e.g. spontaneous abortion, ectopic pregnancy; too much information on risks by healthcare practitioners, or conversely concerns regarding wellbeing dismissed
Dealing with risk	Wants to be seen as a good mother, breastfeeding, accessing help and support, e.g. FNP; participation in antenatal classes, particularly if group organised for teenage mothers	Access to pre-conceptual care; requesting additional screening/diagnostic tests; educating themselves; engaging in a healthy lifestyle; ignoring risks, emotional detachment from pregnancy; emphasis on positive aspects – readiness to parent, problem-solving skills acquired through life experience; religious beliefs and hopes

Table 3.2: Concepts providing risk to pregnancy related to age

---

Activity 3.3   *Critical thinking*

Using the information above, explore and make a list of the psychological and social factors that may influence teenage girls and women of advanced age when booking for antenatal care. Consider where there may be similarities and differences between the two age groups and what you may be able to do as a midwife to address these factors?

How will you demonstrate the **NHS values** (DH, 2013a) in your approach to their care?

How will you use the **6 'Cs' of care** (DH, 2012) to support and guide these women through the emotional and social aspects of childbearing?

The questions raised in this activity are discussed in the text below.

Some of the similarities could include both women feeling anxious but possibly embarrassed, particularly the older woman if surrounded by much younger women within an antenatal clinic setting. Both may fear being judged for becoming pregnant 'at their age' which may lead to a mixture of emotions including shame, pleasure, excitement and joy and possibly regret. Reassuring these women that everyone counts, irrespective of age, and treating all with dignity and respect is an essential element of a midwife's role. Midwives will work in partnership with mothers and their families and other health and social care professionals to improve the lives of mothers and babies. These women may feel 'out of sync' with the majority of women giving birth and have concerns about their ability to be a good parent, perhaps from different perspectives. They may share concerns regarding their ability to manage financially due to lack of employment or access to benefits for teenage girls compared to loss of salary while on maternity leave/returning to part-time work for older women. Midwives should try to understand the priorities, needs, strengths and weakness of women of all ages and afford a level of communication which women understand and feel engaged, so remaining partners in their care. Women's trust will be gained from a midwife who provides a commitment to the quality of care.

In addition pregnant teenagers typical of those cited in the SEU (1999) report may be late booking for antenatal care or conceal their pregnancy. They may feel uncertain about their housing situation, fearing expulsion from the family home due to anger/guilt/shame expressed by parents, which may be exacerbated by a fear of rejection from current relationships with parents/carers/boyfriends. For women of advanced maternal age, the known increased risk of a baby being born with a congenital abnormality may cause pregnancy and birth to be an extremely anxious period possibly aggravated by concern over loss of employment status, financial reward associated with employment combined with social isolation and adjustment to motherhood. In addition the older the woman the more time she has had to accumulate co-morbidities such as hypertension or diabetes, particularly if associated with obesity. On the contrary the older woman may have accessed pre-conceptual care and taken responsibility for promoting her wellbeing, fitness and planned for pregnancy and childbearing.

Activity 3.4 — *Decision-making*

You and your colleague work in a team of midwives providing care in the community and caseload women to provide continuity of care during labour. Using NICE guidance for antenatal care (NICE, 2008), intrapartum care (NICE, 2014a) and postnatal care (NICE, 2014b) plan care for the following women:

1. Bianca is a 16-year-old who lives with her mother and her two siblings who are younger than her. She knows she has missed at least four periods, which are normally regular, by which time she is feeling so scared that she decides to tell her mum. She generally enjoys good health though schoolwork and the pressure of exams do tend to make her feel down and sometimes anxious. She deals with this by smoking, but her mum does not know this.

2. Felicity is a 39-year-old television production engineer who has been trying to conceive with her partner for the last six years. She has had two spontaneous abortions and her last pregnancy ended in an ectopic pregnancy requiring a salpingectomy performed at 7 weeks of pregnancy. Felicity travels 45 minutes each way to work. Due to her obstetric history she has accessed pre-conceptual advice from her practice nurse.

    (a) How will you address biological, social and psychological care needs for these two women in accordance with the guidance offered by NICE?
    (b) What advice and management will be required to promote normality and wellbeing?
    (c) Is any additional care required due to their age and history?

The questions raised in this activity are discussed in the text below.

The lack of antenatal care for Bianca may restrict the ability to access the full range of combined screening tests for congenital abnormalities, particularly if booking occurs after 20 weeks' gestation. It may also compromise the ability to perform other antenatal screening tests and effect appropriate treatment, for example a full blood count to detect haemoglobin level, possible anaemia and instigate oral iron therapy. Determining if the woman is rhesus negative is best performed as early as possible in pregnancy to ensure anti-D immunoglobulin is offered as appropriate at any possible occasion of possible sensitisation. By contrast Felicity is likely to book early due to being anxious and will have opportunity to access all screening in accordance with the NHS Antenatal and Newborn screening timeline (**www.screening. nhs.uk/nhs-timeline**).

Both women may benefit from information on diet and foods to avoid while pregnant, advice on alcohol intake and following carbon monoxide monitoring for both women, Bianca will be offered referral to smoking cessation services. The above advice, combined with a plan of antenatal care reflective of NICE guidance may incorporate additional visits to monitor fetal wellbeing and growth to avoid low birth weight and hopefully preterm birth. If circumstances allow booking may be conducted in the woman's own home and antenatal and breastfeeding classes offered with women of a similar age to facilitate social support in the postnatal period and beyond.

Multi-agency working, particularly for Bianca, and liaison with education services will facilitate her transition back to education with support from a 'care to learn' scheme. Dependent upon the reaction of her mother she may require support from a social worker to access foster care or local authority supported housing services.

Both Bianca and Felicity may be classed as 'consultant-led care' in accordance with local Trust guidance/protocols for care. However care in labour should be provided in accordance with NICE guidance and the use of the RCM evidence-based guidelines for midwifery-led care in labour (RCM, 2012) provides the basis of care that can be offered to all women in labour providing the midwife pays additional attention to any specific needs these women have and refer to a medical practitioner should any deviation from normal arise (NMC, 2009, 2012, 2015).

Both women should have their postnatal care planned holistically around their individual needs. Supporting both women to initiate breastfeeding is an essential skill for a midwife (NMC, 2009). Recognition of the possibility of social isolation for both women and encouragement to attend sessions at Children's Centres such as baby massage may help to alleviate this and mental health problems associated with childbearing. Both women require information and advice on how to recognise that their body has returned to its non-pregnant state with education and advice on contraceptive methods and how to access service provision. Information on infant health and child safety plus handover of care to the health visitor is appropriate for both women, but of particular relevance for teenage mothers due to the high infant mortality rate in this group.

Activity 3.5   *Reflection*

Thinking about your approach to care for Bianca and Felicity, and drawing on your experience of caring for women across the age span, reflect on the following questions:

- Does your communication style need to change when talking to women at either end of the age spectrum? What factors may influence the information you may provide?

- Is care of these women, who may have some additional care requirements, the remit of all midwives or are they better served by specialist midwives who may have additional knowledge and skills to support the needs of these women?

The answers to these questions will depend upon your own experience and reflections, so no answer is provided.

The trend for delayed childbearing looks set to continue for the foreseeable future, which raises the question of how it should be approached from a healthcare perspective. The Royal College of Obstetricians and Gynaecologists (RCOG) released a statement in 2009 declaring that the public should be better informed of the increased risks associated with pregnancy at an advanced maternal age, but that women should also be supported in their choices (RCOG, 2009b). The College makes the point that organisations such as itself, NICE and the Department of Health will have to work together to tackle the challenges of caring for this growing group of women. This could also include the voluntary sector, such as the National Childbirth Trust (NCT).

In many areas of the country the Family Nurse Partnership (FNP) programme, a community-based nurse led intensive home visiting programme for vulnerable first time mothers aged under 20, is being commissioned by NHS England (Local Authorities from April 2015). Within commissioned areas this service is reserved for the most vulnerable under-20-year-old pregnant teenagers and it is crucial that the midwifery service works in tandem with the FNP. This programme is underpinned by research that demonstrates it can improve the health, social and educational outcomes in the short-, medium- and long-term, while providing cost benefits. It aims to support teenagers to:

- have a healthy pregnancy;
- improve their child's health and development;
- plan their own futures and achieve their aspirations.

A family nurse regularly visits at home (every 1–2 weeks) from early in pregnancy until the child is two years old. Home visits usually last between 1 and 1.5 hours. Examples of topics for home visits that can be negotiated by the mother and family nurse include:

- keeping healthy in pregnancy;
- preparing for labour;
- supporting your baby to grow and learn;
- planning to meet life goals.

In trials in America, it has consistently been found to result in:

- improved pregnancy outcomes;
- reduced child abuse and neglect;
- improved school readiness;
- reduced youth crime;
- improved employment for mothers, and fewer subsequent pregnancies with bigger gaps between births.

(FNP, 2015)

Activity 3.6   *Research and evidence-based practice*

Access the Family Nurse Partnership webpage (**http://fnp.nhs.uk**) to read the three case stories of teenage mums from different backgrounds to learn of how their pregnancy and parenting experience was made a positive one. The website also provides access to recent research on this topic. Do any of these cases resonate with women you have cared for? If you were to meet the same situation again, based on reading these stories, would you do anything different?

As this activity is based on your own research, no answer is given at the end of the chapter.

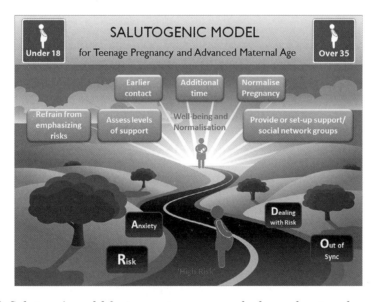

Figure 3.3: Salutogenic model for teenage pregnancy and advanced maternal age (reproduced from Hood, 2014, with permission)

Figure 3.3 shows you what positive care across the age span looks like: it depicts the salutogenic 'road' towards wellbeing and normalisation of pregnancy for teenagers and women of advanced maternal age. It will help you with Activity 3.6, as well as to reflect on this chapter as a whole.

Activity 3.7   *Critical thinking*

To summarise your learning from this chapter use each of the boxes identified as contributing to wellbeing and normalisation of pregnancy; list possible advice and/or action you may take as a midwife to support salutogenesis for teenage or older mums in the antenatal period, for and in labour and during the postnatal period.

	Teenage mums	**Older mums**
Earlier contact		
Additional time		
Normalise pregnancy		
Refrain from emphasising the risks		
Assess levels of support		
Provide or set up support or social network groups		

An answer to this activity is given at the end of the chapter.

(Hood, 2014, with permission)

Completion of this activity will enable you to recognise and fulfil your role as a midwife in normalising a health and wellbeing approach to childbearing for teenagers and older women with continual regard to the requirements of the NMC Standards (NMC, 2009) and NMC Midwives Rules and Standards (NMC, 2012) and The Code of professional conduct (NMC, 2015).

Chapter summary

A midwife's role is to promote and support normality in pregnancy while remaining vigilant to the detection and appropriate referral of any abnormality. Facilitating and guiding women at either end of the age spectrum along the road to normalising pregnancy may be challenging given the significant research and expert opinion that exists to support the concept of increased risks for these age groups, albeit the existence of challenges to these risks. Acknowledgement of what are the risks and how to deal with these may enable the mother and her family to visualise and anticipate a normal pregnancy, with appropriate support from a range of professionals and services. Midwives need to be supported to provide a holistic model of care that focuses on the social and emotional needs of these women as well as their biological needs, to relieve anxiety, raise self-esteem and enable them to feel positive about their pregnancy and future parenting.

The salutogenic 'road' has been mapped in this chapter to signpost midwives to strategies they may use to assist this process. Working in accordance with the NHS values (DH, 2013a) and the vision and strategy to provide compassion in practice through implementation of the 6 Cs of care (DH, 2012) will assist midwives to support women at either end of the age spectrum on their journey through childbearing to achieve the best possible health outcomes.

Activity: brief outline answer

Activity 3.7 Critical thinking [page 54]

You might have completed the box like this:

	Teenage mums	Older mums
Earlier contact	This group may need support to recognise possibility of pregnancy, testing and early diagnosis with encouragement to book for antenatal care by 10 weeks of pregnancy and therefore access screening programmes to promote maternal health and fetal wellbeing. Advised to start folic acid 400 micrograms as soon as possible.	These mums will be able to access combined screening test for Down's syndrome, including nuchal translucency. They may have accessed pre-conceptual care and taken folic acid, 400 micrograms for 3 months prior to conception, plus first 3 months of pregnancy.
Additional time	Make a longer appointment time for antenatal/postnatal visit. Conduct visits in the woman's home. Offer more frequent visits rather than minimum recommended by NICE (2015).	Allay fears and address anxiety related to physical recovery from pregnancy and labour and the wellbeing of the fetus. Offer more frequent visits rather than minimum recommended by NICE (2015).
Normalise pregnancy	Encourage activities that will keep the woman feeling well. Specific health promotion on components of a healthy diet, alcohol intake, smoking cessation, exercise. Availability of specialist midwives with specific skills and ability to offer longer appointment times can support this.	Provide an individualised holistic approach to health and wellbeing throughout pregnancy – advice on weight gain, exercise, adjustment to motherhood. Discuss place of delivery.
Refrain from emphasising the risks	Emphasise the positive; health promotion, general health and wellbeing. How to recognise and promote wellbeing e.g. support for breastfeeding. Mindfulness to focus on the present.	Avoid labels such as 'high risk' or 'elderly primip'. Emphasise maintenance of good health through diet, exercise and lifestyle management, e.g. reduce alcohol intake.

	Teenage mums	**Older mums**
Assess levels of support	Enquire about family support, friends and peers. What help will be needed to continue their education. Refer to social services if assistance with finance and housing needed.	Consider the social capital available – may have limited social networks if spent years working full time. Consider if extended family or friends in surrounding area.
Provide or set up support or social network groups	Are there enough teenage mums to run an antenatal class or breastfeeding support group for this age group? This may become a postnatal support group with long lasting friendships and social support.	Encourage attendance at antenatal preparation/hypno-birthing/NCT/ baby massage classes. Liaise with health visitor colleagues to provide access to local support groups.

N.B. Note similarity of approach in both age groups.

Further reading

Hunter, L. (2013) Discourses of teenage motherhood: finding a framework that enables provision of appropriate support. Part 1: Risk discourses and the shortcomings of the Teenage Pregnancy Strategy. *Essentially MIDIRS*, 4 (3): 32–37 and Part 2: Situational and developmental perspectives. *Essentially MIDIRS*, 4 (4): 32–37.

Kenyon, A.P. (2010) Effect of age on maternal and fetal outcomes. *British Journal of Midwifery*, 18 (6): 358–362.

Social Exclusion Unit [SEU] (1999) *Teenage Pregnancy*. London: The Stationery Office. **http:// dera.ioe.ac.uk/15086/1/teenage-pregnancy.pdf**

Chapter 4
Women who have communication challenges

Sam Chenery-Morris

 NMC Standards for Pre-registration Midwifery Education

This chapter will address the following competencies:

Domain: Effective midwifery practice

Communicate effectively with women and their families throughout the pre-conception, antenatal, intrapartum and postnatal periods. Communication will include:

- Listening to the woman and helping them identify their feelings and anxieties about their pregnancies, the birth and related changes to themselves and their lives.
- Enabling women to think about their feelings.
- Enabling women to make informed choices about their health and healthcare.
- Actively encouraging women to think about their own health and the health of their babies and families and how this can be improved.
- Communicating with women throughout their pregnancy, labour and the period following birth.

Care for, monitor and support women during labour and monitor the condition of the fetus, supporting spontaneous births. This will include:

- Communicating with women throughout and supporting them through the experience.
- Ensuring that the care is sensitive to individual women's culture and preferences.
- Using appropriate clinical and technical means to monitor the condition of the mother and fetus.
- Providing appropriate pain management.
- Providing appropriate care to women once they have given birth.

Domain: Achieving quality care through evaluation and research

Apply relevant knowledge to the midwife's own practice in structured ways which are capable of evaluation. This will include:

- Critical appraisal of knowledge and research evidence.
- Critical appraisal of midwife's own practice.
- Gaining feedback from women and their families and appropriately applying this to practice.
- Disseminating critically appraised good practice.

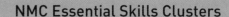

NMC Essential Skills Clusters

This chapter will address the following ESCs:

Cluster: Communication

Women can trust/expect a newly registered midwife to:

1. Be attentive and share information that is clear, accurate and meaningful at a level which women, their partners and family can understand.
7. Provide care that is delivered in a warm, sensitive and compassionate way.

Cluster: Initial consultation between the woman and the midwife

Complete an initial consultation accurately ensuring the women are at the centre of care.

Chapter aims

After reading this chapter you will be able to:

- understand the complexity of issues that act as barriers for women with communication difficulties in accessing and attending appointments;
- consider areas of best practice and embed these into your practice;
- ensure effective communication is available for all women so each woman can make informed decisions and be satisfied in their care.

Introduction

This chapter will consider the issues facing women who are recent migrants, asylum seekers or refugees. Many of these women will face communication challenges with healthcare professionals. The challenges are not solely related to their English language fluency. Initially this chapter will consider ethnicity and the barriers facing recent migrant women. The principles of good practice for interpreting services will be stated, but access to services, understanding the UK healthcare system and financial difficulties will also be addressed. This will give you the opportunity to consider the challenges many of these women face and consider how you the individual can make a difference and whether there is a lack of suitable resources in your area for its demographics.

We continue with the underlying theme of the previous chapters, that communication between you, the midwife, and the woman is paramount. The woman and her family should be at the centre of any decisions made. To facilitate this you and the woman must be able to communicate. During this chapter there will be opportunities to consider your own knowledge and attitude towards women with complex social factors, including limited English language or communication skills, and possibly change your thinking. The reason for these activities is to help you develop an insight into how you might develop your own practice and achieve quality care through personal and professional evaluation and research. At present the needs of women who have communication barriers are diverse and no one method or model of communication can work for all women, so the evidence for how best to communicate with women with language barriers is limited.

What is known is the demographics of the UK have changed dramatically over the last few decades. While the exact numbers of migrant pregnant women in the UK are not known, the latest Office for National Statistics report shows a quarter of births (25.9%) in 2011 were to mothers born outside the UK (Zumpe *et al.*, 2012). Of course many of these women will have no language barrier, but some will. In 2011, there were 808,000 births in the UK, of these 196,000 births were to non-UK born women. This is an increase of 9% in the last decade, since 2001.

First, let's consider the terminology.

Activity 4.1   *Critical thinking*

With a colleague consider what the terms recent migrant, asylum seeker and refugee mean.

An answer is given at the end of this chapter.

While the three terms above have specific meanings, there are several other terms used when considering ethnicity. When a literature review looked at increased risk of maternal death among ethnic minority women in the UK the terminology used in research papers was found to be varied (Ameh and van den Broek, 2008).

Terminology	Description
Ethnic minority groups	Ethnic group other than White British women
Non-White groups	Groups other than White British
Immigrant women	Women born outside the UK
Non-English speaking women	Women who do not speak English
Migrant women	Includes refugees, asylum seekers and recently arrived women
Travellers	Includes gypsy population and population with no fixed abode

Table 4.1: Defining terminology (Ameh and van den Broek, 2008)

Understanding ethnicity

To understand women's needs we need to explore the term ethnicity. Ethnicity is usually thought to encompass socially constructed differences between groups of people who share common ancestry, language, religion, geographical territory and customs. Within the UK, there are four countries, two official languages (English and Welsh) and minority ethnic groups. The differences between the ethnic groups are as diverse as the differences between the White populations; to explain this let's look at the latest UK census data. This census was undertaken on 27 March 2011, the results of statistics are available on the census website and these statistics relate to England and Wales only on this date.

	All persons	Males	Females
All categories: Ethnic group	56,075,912	27,573,376	28,502,536
White: Total	48,209,395	23,630,918	24,578,477
English/Welsh/Scottish/ Northern Irish/British	45,134,686	22,167,807	22,966,879
Irish	531,087	254,427	276,660
Gypsy or Irish Traveller	57,680	28,596	29,084
Other White	2,485,942	1,180,088	1,305,854
Mixed/multiple ethnic group: Total	1,224,400	611,533	612,867
White and Black Caribbean	426,715	211,605	215,110
White and Black African	165,974	82,995	82,979
White and Asian	341,727	175,686	166,041
Other Mixed	289,984	141,247	148,737
Asian/Asian British: Total	4,213,531	2,120,157	2,093,374
Indian	1,412,958	719,920	693,038
Pakistani	1,124,511	576,215	548,296
Bangladeshi	447,201	230,871	216,330
Chinese	393,141	186,028	207,113
Other Asian	835,720	407,123	428,597
Black/African/Caribbean/ Black British: Total	1,864,890	898,200	966,690
African	989,628	479,799	509,829
Caribbean	594,825	276,937	317,888

Other Black	280,437	141,464	138,973
Other ethnic group: Total	563,696	312,568	251,128
Arab	230,600	134,143	96,457
Any other ethnic group	333,096	178,425	154,671

Table 4.2: Demographic statistics from the England and Wales census (ONS, 2011)

From the list of statistics presented above you will see that ethnicity of England and Wales in 2011, when these figures were taken, is diverse. There are problems with census data, since the data asks for racial categories (Black or White) and nationalities, or geographical areas (African, Bangladeshi, Chinese, Indian, etc.). Clearly being Indian is not an ethnicity, by this we mean, India is a huge country populated by different ethnic communities itself, but when understood by the UK census the people from India are considered one group. Remember too that someone can be British and Black, or Indian. Similarly being White does not mean that someone is from a majority population or British. Migrant women are different from UK born ethnic minorities. There are substantial proportions of mothers of Black Caribbean, Indian, Pakistani ethnic origin, who were themselves born in the UK.

If we look at the whole population, 56 million people, the majority (85%) are White (48 million people). But within the White category there are still differences and being White is not unproblematic nor does it mean 'non-ethnic' majority status, as we will see. 45 million people or 80% said they were British, English, Scottish, Welsh and/or of Northern Irish ethnicity (remembering you can be both British and English at the same time or Welsh and Scottish). This leaves 3 million other White people within the UK. Three other categories of White were recorded on the census for the first time. In the 2001 census White was not broken down into different White ethnicities; at that time 92.1% of the population was White.

Now the other White categories include Irish (approx 530,000 people or 1%), from the Republic of Ireland (not Northern Ireland), Gypsy or Irish Traveller (approx 57,000 people or 0.1%) and other White groups (2.5 million people or 4.5%). Being a Gypsy or Irish Traveller is clearly an ethnic minority in the UK despite being of a White racial category and of the 4.5% of people who are other White groups, the differences between them and their ethnicity is also likely to be huge.

If we look at the numbers of people defined as Indian now we will see 1.4 million people or 2.5% of the UK population are Indian, but there will be many different ethnic groups within those figures. This exploration of the UK demographics shows that being a minority ethnic group is not synonymous with being Black or Asian, as there are minority ethnic groups within the White populations as well and each group will have a particular culture, shared ancestry, language, religion and customs. As a midwife, while it is helpful to have some understanding of different ethnic groups, the most important aspect of your role is not to assume you know what certain types of people want or need or to stereotype ethnic groups. The essence of women-centred individual care is paramount. To know what a woman wants, whatever her ethnicity, you have to communicate with her.

Migration statistics

While the census tells us how many people are living in the UK on a given day every decade, it does not tell us how many people have migrated to the UK in a given year. Women living in the UK who were born abroad originate from a wide variety of countries. Over 200 different maternal countries of birth were recorded on birth registrations in the UK in 2011. From the Office for National Statistics, it is known that the greatest number of women coming to the UK to have babies in 2011 were from Poland. There were 23,000 births from these women in all four countries of the UK (Zumpe *et al.*, 2012). The top 10 countries are listed below with the number of births in thousands.

Position	Country of maternal birth	Thousands
1	Poland	23.0
2	Pakistan	19.2
3	India	15.5
4	Bangladesh	8.5
5	Nigeria	7.9
6	Somalia	5.7
7	Germany	5.6
8	South Africa	4.8
9	Lithuania	4.2
10	China	4.1

Table 4.3: Top 10 countries of birth for non-UK born mothers of live births in the UK, 2011 (Zumpe et al., 2012)

What this table tells us is for every 100 births to women born abroad, 12 mothers would have been born in Poland, 10 in Pakistan and 8 in India. The rest of the top 10 would account for another 20 mothers, with the other 50 from other recorded countries (Zumpe *et al.*, 2012). While statistics tell us where the women were born, this is not the whole picture and care must be taken when considering these statistics, since a woman may not have been born in the UK but she may be a British National, this is particularly true for the country of birth for Germany, since many women born there were to families serving in the UK armed forces. Similarly a woman who was born in South Africa may be from another country. Some of these women may face no language barriers at all, others may experience difficulties accessing healthcare and communicating in English.

Your experience of providing care for migrant women will depend on where you are learning to be a midwife and where you work when you are qualified, as there are great variations within the UK. The proportion of births to women born outside the UK ranged from 11% in Wales to 57% in London in 2011 (Zumpe *et al.*, 2012).

The most common reason for migrating long-term to the UK is to study (42% in 2010), followed by work, and then accompanying/joining family members. Just 4% of net migration to the UK is to asylum applicants and their dependents, despite what you might believe in the media representation. The women who migrate to the UK to study, work or accompany their family members will clearly have different needs from the asylum-seeking women. Understanding the UK system, however, and knowing how to access services and language barriers may be common to many of these women.

It is not just communication challenges that these women face; the maternal health outcomes and infant mortality is significantly worse for migrant women than for the rest of the UK population (Jayaweera and Quigley, 2010). Evidence suggests that some of this is preventable since migrant health is often good when they arrive in the UK. Thus this chapter will look at reasons for the differences and what you can do to help reduce the statistics for these women and improve their experiences.

Understanding the extent of the problem

The health outcomes of recent migrant women in the UK are not all as good as the native population. Inequality in health is highlighted by the number of women in the UK who died in the Saving Mother's Lives (CMACE, 2011) report. Twenty-eight women were of Black African ethnicity in the three years (2006–2008). Of these women, 9 were UK citizens but the other 19 had recently arrived in the UK. Several newly arrived Asian brides who could not speak English also died and women from EU countries new to the UK too. The statistics from this report are shocking: for White women there is an estimated 80 cases of severe maternal morbidity per 100,000 maternities, whereas for women from Black or other minority ethnic groups this figure is 126 cases per 100,000 maternities (CMACE, 2011). In the 2009–2012 report (Knight *et al.*, 2014) a third of the women who died were born outside the UK; the average length of time they had lived in the UK was for 4 years (range from 1 month to 21 years). The majority of women who died were Asian or African (70%), although some were from Poland and other countries. Women born outside the UK were significantly more likely to die than those born in the UK, with Nigerian women most at risk.

Of course, not all Black women or those from minority ethnic groups have communication challenges; many women speak English, but the population risk ratio is significantly higher than that for White women, even after adjustments are made for differences in age, socioeconomic and smoking status, obesity and parity.

Reasons for these shocking statistics are multifactoral. Recently arrived migrants may have comparatively poor overall health and underlying medical conditions which may be undiagnosed and this contributes to their higher maternal morbidity and mortality rates, but many have good health. Cultural factors such as female genital mutilation or the psychological effects of leaving a home country and friends and family behind may also impact upon health. Fears about immigration status and language difficulties also contribute to poor maternal health. Non-UK born Black and minority ethnic women are less likely to be offered antenatal care than UK born White women (Redshaw *et al.*, 2007). The same group of women reported less access to care options and poor health postnatally. Other reasons for inequalities in maternal health outcomes consider structural barriers to good health, such as poor housing, inadequate financial resources, migrants lacking knowledge of access and uptake of screening immunisation and inadequate professional support, including accessing language support (Johnson, 2006).

Barriers migrant women face in accessing maternity services

In the UK the aim is for women to meet their midwife early in the pregnancy, ideally by 10 weeks' gestation (NICE, 2008). However, for different groups of women there are different barriers to meeting this ideal. For instance a recent migrant may not have this early philosophy of care in their home country, so see no need to access maternity services early in the UK. Some women may not realise there are interpreting services to meet their needs and see their lack

Service barriers reported by women	Personal reasons which act as barriers reported by women	Barriers reported by providers
Language – lack of interpreters, use of colloquialisms	Not understanding the healthcare system and how to access it	Language
Discrimination, racism towards immigrants and non-English speakers	Lack of social network	Lack of availability of suitable interpreters, especially for emergencies, out of hours and unbooked appointments
	Misunderstanding dates and times of appointments	
Lack of continuity of carer	Not understanding the purpose of antenatal classes, diagnostic tests	Unfamiliarity of healthcare system, what to expect and how to use it
Not told about antenatal education		Ethnic minority women do not conform to rules – use emergency services instead of clinics, can be demanding expecting healthcare to live up to standards in their home country
Refused registration with a GP	Women experiencing depression, fear, anxiety or other personal problems	
Lack of transport	Financial	
Inconvenient time of antenatal clinic	Lack of childcare	
No directing agencies	Fear of immigration services	Lack of knowledge of cultural and religious differences
Lack of cultural sensitivity among providers	Dispersement policies for women with asylum seeker/ refugee status	Negative attitude towards women from ethnic minorities
Negative attitude of healthcare professionals	Lack of assertiveness in dealing with healthcare system	Lack of continuity of carer
		Pressures and difficulties arising from immigration status

Table 4.4: Barriers for women with little or no English (reproduced from NICE, 2010a, p87)

of English fluency as a barrier to accessing healthcare generally. Speaking English and understanding medical terms are quite different. Migrant women may have experienced negative healthcare attitudes before and this deters them from seeking midwifery care. NICE (2010a) compiled a table of barriers for recent migrants, refugees, asylum seekers and women with little or no English (see Table 4.4).

Activity 4.2 — *Communication*

Look at Table 4.4 and consider if there are aspects of professional behaviour you may have witnessed that could be improved? Consider your duty in becoming and being a professional.

An outline answer, suggesting areas you may have noticed and ideas to improve professional practice, is given at the end of the chapter.

Professional attitudes and behaviours of healthcare staff matter to all service users. Migrant women have reported negative attitude of healthcare professionals and discrimination or racism towards them and their lack of English language as barriers to accessing healthcare (NICE, 2010a). Once women do access services, it is important that they are treated with respect and that their communication barriers are resolved to adequately assess the care needs of each individual, to provide education about the pregnancy and birth but also the healthcare system so these women can make informed choices about all aspects of their care.

It is a legal requirement to ensure that patients whose first language is not English, should be provided access to an appropriate communication support service. The correct terminology used when one transfers ideas orally or by the use of gestures from one language to another is interpreting. This refers to either oral English language into British Sign Language or oral English language into another language, whether that is Spanish, Israeli or any other language. When writing is used, from written English to another language, the term used is translation.

The reason for having an appropriate communication service is to protect the woman. Having a family member or friend interpret may seem an innocent practice until you consider what may go wrong with this practice.

Activity 4.3 — *Critical thinking*

Consider the following cases:

Alma is at her antenatal appointment with her mother interpreting for her. The midwife asks if she is worried about her personal relationships, wellbeing or safety.

Freida is accompanied by her 14-year-old daughter who interprets for her. The midwife asks about Freida's previous medical and obstetric history.

continued ...

---

continued . . .

> Meena is accompanied by her husband; she has limited understanding of English. When informed about screening options, her husband says without asking Meena that they do not require screening.
>
> With a colleague determine the possible consequences within these scenarios and others you may have come across.
>
> *Some possible answers are given at the end of the chapter.*

From the exercise you can see that using family members or friends for interpreting is highly inappropriate and lends itself to a degree of risk. These risks include patient confidentiality, lack of disclosure of risk factors, lack of informed consent and possible care that is determined by the relative's values as opposed to the woman's.

Interpreting is a professional skill which requires appropriate and effective use; we have already mentioned the terminology which is specific to midwifery. Trained interpreters are skilled at understanding the terminology and relaying this to women in their own language, so their preferences can be heard. It is not professionally and ethically acceptable to use children (under 16) as interpreters. Health professionals must therefore identify patients' communication needs, where possible, on initial contact and document these in the patients' notes. This will facilitate a proactive response to meet individual need. Check the woman's maternity notes for specific communication needs. If you have any difficulty in communicating fully with a patient, it is a requirement for you to arrange for a suitable interpreter through the Trust interpreting services. Interpreters should be used for all planned admissions, assessments, clinical consultations, informed consent and discharge.

So, the general principles of caring for women with communication challenges while in your care is that you provide appropriate resources to meet their communication need. For women who have limited English language an interpreter is also a necessity.

Role of the interpreter

The role of the interpreter is to interpret accurately what is said, without anything being added, omitted or changed. Professional interpreters will respect confidentiality at all times and not seek advantage of any information disclosed during the interview. Their code of conduct states they will act in an impartial and professional manner and be non-judgemental. They will interpret without giving advice or reaction to the conversation. They will disclose immediately if they are having difficulties with dialect or medical terminology, or if the patient is known or related to them.

The interpreter will only intervene to seek clarification; to point out if someone has not understood something; or to identify any cultural misunderstanding.

Working effectively with interpreters requires thought and planning. Health professionals working in busy clinics and ward environments may have their own preferred ways of working, therefore may be unprepared for the dynamics and complexity of a three or four way dialogue. It is important to recognise that some preparatory work can be useful.

When booking an interpreter the following procedure should be allowed:

- Give the interpreter adequate notice: a minimum 24 hours unless it is an emergency.
- Provide patient information to the interpreter on pertinent issues, e.g. a patient's mental state or a patient's inability to communicate verbally.
- Allow enough time for the interview – twice as long as an interview without an interpreter.
- Explanations of cultural perceptions and backgrounds may be required.
- Indicate how long the session is likely to run.
- Ensure that the interpreter and the patient speak the same language and dialect.
- Match the gender of interpreter and patient if appropriate.
- Explain the nature of the interview.

During the interview

- Allow time for introductions and for the interpreter to develop a rapport with the patient and to explain the interpreter's role as being there to give an impartial, complete, accurate and confidential interpretation of everything that is said by everyone present in the room.
- Be aware of the seating arrangement, to ensure that the healthcare professional and the interpreter face the patient directly. Try to speak directly to the patient, i.e. 'What is your name?' rather than 'Will you ask her what her name is?' Also ask directly if you are not sure of relevant culture based facts or perceptions. Speak in clear, short sentences with pauses in between for the interpreter to interpret what you are saying.
- Avoid jargon, abbreviations and specialist terminology wherever possible, letting the interpreter interrupt you if they need to clarify something. Be aware that the woman when speaking may not leave pauses for the interpreter and that the interpreter may give you a summary – ask interpreter for a more detailed version of what was said.
- Behave as you would if you shared the same language, recognising and respecting individual backgrounds. Conduct all the interview yourself. Do not ask the interpreter to fill in a form or explain a procedure. The interpreter is not qualified to look for relevant information or to process information received.

At the end of the interview

- Check that the patient has understood everything. Summarise what has been decided and explain the next practical steps to be taken – when, where and how. Arrange for the appointment while the interpreter is there.
- Ask if there is anything else the patient would like to know. If not recorded before then enter the patient's communication need in the notes.

Now you have the principles of best practice for interpreting, undertake Activity 4.4 to see what is available in your local area.

Activity 4.4   *Research and evidence-based practice*

Look on your hospital or community Trust intranet and access the communication or interpretation and translation policy. It will state which services are offered in your area and should be responsive to the changing demographics of your local area.

There is an NHS Trust policy provided at the end of this chapter; see how this compares to your findings. Two case studies follow that show how different areas offer different services depending on their clientele.

Now you have considered communication attitudes and interpretation services we will look at a scenario to bring together the barriers migrant women face and aspects of midwifery care.

Scenario 1

A primigravid woman, Justyna, is transferred from the accident and emergency unit to the maternity assessment unit. She is 32 weeks' pregnant and has not yet been seen by a midwife; she presents with a headache and feeling unwell. Justyna is Polish, and she is a qualified teacher but working as a class-room assistant as she develops her English language skills.

What are your initial thoughts on this scenario?

If we refer back to Table 4.4, outlining barriers reported by recent migrants and providers of care to accessing maternity services, we can see Justyna's presentation to A and E is not uncommon. Clearly we cannot say why Justyna did not schedule an appointment prior to her emergency presentation, but it is likely that some of the factors such as lack of knowledge about the UK system or her working pattern may have been barriers to her accessing maternity care sooner.

Justyna is an educated woman with limited English language skills. Her presentation at A and E with a headache and feeling unwell may be a symptom of raised blood pressure; while this can be treated there are many aspects of midwifery care that Justyna has missed and communicating to her now is important, so she understands what the present plan of care is and when next to be seen. So your priority now, as Justyna's midwife, is to aid effective communication with her. You will need an interpreter to ensure Justyna fully understands all her care options. All information should be accessible to women who do not speak English (NICE, 2008). Information can be given in audiovisual forms or via touch screen technologies; whilst these should be supported by written information, the first step is clearly communicating with Justyna now.

If it is not possible to access an interpreter now, digital technologies and the internet can be used to ensure Justyna gets the information in her first language.

Activity 4.5   *Research and evidence-based practice*

With a fellow student, visit the following websites and see what information is available and in which languages:

www.babycentre.co.uk/a1018094/translated-articles

www.nct.org.uk/professional/diversity-and-access/supporting-parents-black-and-minority-ethnic-groups-refugees-and-4

There are no suggested answers at the end of this chapter but it is hoped that you will access these resources when required.

As you have seen from the above activity there are many leaflets available on aspects of maternity care in various languages. This leaflet could be printed for Justyna: **www.babycentre.co.uk/a1018397/pregnancy-symptoms-you-should-never-ignore**

Your Trust may have some specific information sheets in the languages frequently encountered by its demographic populations; see if you can access those too, so you have a repertoire to refer to.

There are other internet based resources, especially when interpreting services are not available, such as during unscheduled appointments such as the onset of spontaneous labour. The Obstetric Anaesthetists' Association has launched a smartphone application for mothers to be in 35 different languages. Because this is an app, no internet connection is required and many women have smartphones, so they can use this resource during labour. The languages include Urdu, Hindi, Bengali, Somali, Mandarin, French, Polish, Punjabi, Gujarati and Cantonese. The app includes useful phrases which can aid communication between midwives, doctors and women. There are pain relief options with their associated risks and benefits, so women can make informed choices about these.

While the internet and interpreting services are great when women access maternity services, we still need to consider reasons why migrant women may not access local services. First of all undertake the next activity to see what services there are in your local area.

Activity 4.6   *Research and evidence-based practice*

With a colleague, can you list clinics and resources in your local area which may be specific to migrant populations or generic for all pregnant women?

There are no answers at the end of this chapter as each area will have its own ethnic diversity and resources but the next paragraphs may cover some of the aspects you discussed.

Considering the resources available in your local area is key to improving the integration of migrant women into the UK and their pregnancy outcomes (Bollini *et al.*, 2009). Routine ante-natal midwifery care may be offered in Children's Centres or local GP clinics. Consider the populations that these centres support. These may be within walking distance for some women but others will need to take public transport or drive to access them. If the clinic appointments clash with school or nursery start and finish times this may be a barrier for some women in access-ing routine antenatal care. Combine the dilemma of a woman's older child or children missing school as they cannot be in two places at once and undertaking one or more bus journeys to attend a clinic and you can see why women who may not understand the need for routine ante-natal appointments may not prioritise their visits. Even if they do attend the clinic appointment they meet a different midwife each time. This lack of continuity is a barrier to their continuation. Of course these decisions and issues are faced by all women, but the barrier for migrant women is further complicated. When they attend the clinic if the interpreter is not already booked or cancels at the last minute they are left with an inadequate consultation. This is just the routine appointments. Migrant and most minority ethnic mothers are significantly less likely to have antenatal care or attend antenatal classes (Jayaweera and Quigley, 2010).

There may be simple solutions to these barriers such as drop in clinics, where an appointment is not needed, yet a midwife is present during specific times that may be more convenient to many women, not just migrant women. But communicating how these services work has to be a prior-ity so all women can choose to access the most convenient care. Similarly another clinic might be on a more convenient bus route and this may be preferred. But to know these preferences the midwife has to communicate with the woman to find out her personal circumstances and any difficulties she may have.

Now consider are there any specific groups or activities for social support for different groups in your area, such as antenatal education in Polish, Urdu or Hindi. Are there opportunities for women to meet other pregnant or new mothers who also speak their language, as this can increase their social support networks? Could these be implemented? Perhaps there are bilingual midwives working in your Trust who could facilitate these. The inequalities in migrant pregnancy outcome in the UK can be improved, according to Bollini *et al.* (2009). A more active attitude in recognising difference in individuals and implementing effective interventions to meet their needs will help reduce this inequality.

Now you have considered access to resources, we will return to another barrier from Table 4.4, that of financial barriers that affect women's access to maternity services. Migrant women who come to the UK may have adequate financial resources, compared to those who come to study who may have limited funds. The group of women who face the greatest financial challenges are asylum-seeking women.

Asylum-seeking women

Understanding the legal status of the women in your care will help you know what services they are eligible for. A report (Beecher Bryant, 2011) compiled for Maternity Action, a national charity working to challenge inequality and promote wellbeing for all pregnant women, found many midwives reported confusion around the rights and entitlements of asylum-seeking women. The Department of Health Migrant Friendly Maternity Services (2010) compiled a table of the differences in financial support and benefits available to women of different legal status.

Single British woman	Single asylum seeker	Single failed asylum seeker
Unemployed	Not allowed to work	Not allowed to work
Support throughout pregnancy	Support throughout pregnancy	Support from 32 weeks
£57.35 for women aged 16–24 £72.40 for women over 25 years	£36.62 per week if over 18 + £3 per week for pregnancy	£35.39 per week on a payment card (plus an additional £3 per week from 34 weeks)
£690 maternity grants	£300 maternity grant, usually obtained after birth	£250 maternity grant in vouchers. Usually obtained after birth
Housing assistance	No choice of accommodation, bills paid	No choice of accommodation, bills paid
Free healthcare	Free healthcare	Free primary healthcare (where able to register with a GP), free prescriptions. Charged for secondary healthcare
Free Healthy Start vitamins	No access to Healthy Start vitamins	No access to Healthy Start vitamins

Table 4.5: Financial support and benefits available to different groups of pregnant women (updated from Department of Health, 2010, Migrant Friendly Maternity Services, p36)

Asylum seekers are often portrayed negatively in the UK with the media suggesting they come to the UK for its generous benefit system and National Health Service (Haith-Cooper and Bradshaw, 2013). Once in the UK, pregnant asylum seekers have many barriers to their care, asylum status and access to health, including poor care experiences from health professionals. Evidence suggests that some midwives may demonstrate unprofessional attitudes, rudeness and racism reflected in the media to these women. Student midwives too are influenced by the media and their mentor and can mirror poor attitudes which do not align to woman-centred care. There was evidence of conversations about asylum seekers as being different and with criminal persuasion (Haith-Cooper and Bradshaw, 2013). While some people in the UK may believe this, most people who seek asylum in the UK are fleeing war, rape and other atrocities. It is worth being reminded that asylum applicants and their dependents comprised an estimated 4% of net migration in 2010.

Case study

Fatima has recently arrived from Rwanda. It is her third pregnancy and she is an asylum seeker. She is scheduled for a booking appointment this morning. When your mentor looks at the antenatal appointment schedule she says, 'She'll be a late booker and probably have HIV.'

The midwife is demonstrating an unprofessional attitude towards Fatima's situation. The language the midwife is using is judgemental. The midwife has not yet met Fatima yet she assumes she will be more than 10 weeks' gestation and have an infectious disease. This stereotyped attitude is not woman-focused and will probably be felt by Fatima in how the midwife communicates with her.

Consider instead if the midwife said to you, 'This woman is likely to have fled from the war in her country where rape is a common weapon used against women. She will be living here in the UK on less than £40 per week, and considers herself lucky to be safe despite missing her family back at home.'

Being exposed to these attitudes will shape the midwife you become, especially if you follow the practice of the first example yourself, without perhaps realising what you are saying. During your university learning there may be an opportunity to think about how midwives talk about different groups of women and you may have the opportunity to think about the difficulties these women have experienced and how resilient they are. Your own previous thoughts, often influenced by your family and the media, about migrant women or asylum seekers may be challenged. Reading the work of Haith-Cooper and Bradshaw may also help you see the way language around asylum affects other student midwives and how education can help alter this to a more positive attitude.

To summarise, the main difficulties women who have recently migrated to the UK face is access to effective communication for their care. The barriers to this include lack of interpreting services, lack of local specific services which meet their needs and staff who are not empathetic of their specific barriers.

As a student midwife and then a qualified practitioner there are a number of areas you may need further training on now and in the future to better understand and then meet specific migrant women's needs. These include specific health needs of women recently arrived in the UK who may have female genital mutilation (FGM) or HIV. HIV and FGM are addressed in the sexual health chapter of this book. You may need to know social, religious and psychological needs of these women, and knowledge of government policies on access and entitlement to care. Knowing the demographics of the women in your area is a start, as your Trust will probably have specialised services to meet their needs; if not you will need to read research articles and government websites for the latest evidence and policy to support women in your care. One of the best ways of understanding women's individual needs is to ask them directly, whether this is with the services of an interpreter, in English or their native language if you speak it.

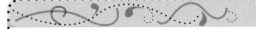

Chapter summary

This chapter introduced the care of the woman and her family when you the midwife do not speak the same language as the woman. It may be that the woman has limited understanding or spoken English. The demographics of the UK have changed immensely in the last two decades and we, as midwives, must use good practices to ensure that these women receive excellent individualised care that meets their needs. This includes full booking interviews to ensure that appropriate referrals are made during the pregnancy which have in the past not been undertaken thoroughly and have contributed to morbidity and mortality in women who do not speak English. Good quality intrapartum care and postnatal services aimed to meet differing women's needs. Communication is at the heart of good effective midwifery care and services are available to communicate with all women. A non-judgemental attitude is also required. As a student and then a qualified midwife you must ensure you know what these services are and access them in a timely manner to meet *all* women's needs.

Activities: brief outline answers

Activity 4.1 Critical thinking [page 59]

Migrant

Someone who migrates from their country to live in the UK.

Asylum seekers

- Someone who has fled from their country because of fear of persecution and has asked for protection in another country.
- Someone who is awaiting a decision on their claim for asylum from the Home Office.
- Not allowed to work or claim mainstream benefits.
- £35 a week and somewhere (no choice) to live.

Refugee

- Someone whose asylum claim has been successful. Has the right to remain in the UK.
- Can work and/or claim mainstream benefits

UN Convention 1951

- Defines refugees as persons who are outside their country and cannot return owing to a well-founded fear of **persecution** because of their **race, religion, nationality, political opinion or membership of a particular social group.**

Activity 4.2 Communication [page 65]

There are aspects within the table that do not meet the NMC (2008) Code of practice. For instance the Code states that you should treat people with respect and must not discriminate in any way. The table of barriers says women have experienced a negative attitude from staff; this is unacceptable. Occasionally you may need to challenge other professionals' opinions, if they are disrespectful or discriminating in their attitudes or care practices. Whilst this is incredibly difficult as a student, your mentor or lecturer will be able to support you. Similarly, as a professional you have a duty to remain knowledgeable and up to date – knowing and understanding cultural or religious differences, especially if there is a particular group in your area of care, is your responsibility.

Activity 4.3 Critical thinking [page 65]

Alma may not disclose if she is experiencing domestic abuse in front of her mother. It is hard enough for women to disclose to healthcare professionals without having to say this through a family member. Similarly the midwife may not ask the question as Alma's mother is present, so she has no opportunity to answer.

Freida may not want her daughter to know about her medical or obstetric history and may therefore not say if she has had a late termination or previous stillborn baby. While this history may not be important if she is rhesus negative and did not receive anti-D following these events it may have real consequences for this pregnancy.

Meena may choose to have more information regarding screening options available to her and her husband. While this may not alter their final decision, not having all the information limits their ability to consent or decline the care option. Alternatively Meena may have a different opinion altogether and would positively like screening, yet she has not had the opportunity to express this choice.

Activity 4.4 Research and evidence-based practice [page 68]

Sample answer from one Trust website

According to the Heart of England NHS Trust website, the following services are available (**www.heartofengland. nhs.uk/wp-content/uploads/Interpreting-and-Translation-Services-Operational-Policy-20112.pdf**):

The Trust interpreting service covers five languages for face to face episodes in Mirpuri, Punjabi, Urdu, Sylheti and Bengali languages.

The Trust written translation service covers two languages for producing patient information in Urdu and Bengali languages.

Language Line – a telephone based interpreting service covering over 100 languages is currently available in three Directorates.

BILCS Interpreting Booking Service provided by Heart of Birmingham Primary Care Trust (Teaching) covers all languages including British Sign Language.

Interpreting agencies which can provide interpreting services in a variety of languages including British Sign Language.

Further reading

All of the below are essential documents that support your care decisions. During the course of your training it is a good idea to read these so you can provide contemporary midwifery care that meets the needs of the UK's diverse population.

NICE (2010) *Pregnant Women with Complex Social Factors.* Chapter 5, Women who are recent migrants, asylum seekers or refugees and women who have difficulties reading or speaking English.

RCN (2009) *Pregnancy and Disability RCN Guidance for Nurses and Midwives.* London: RCN Publishing.

The following textbooks offer further reading:

Richards, Y. (2007) *Challenges for Midwives.* London: Quay Books.

Especially chapters on Midwives and Travellers, Services for women with disabilities, Supporting infant feeding in the Bangladeshi community and Volunteers and users' views of a postnatal listening service for minority ethnic women.

Taylor, S. and Field, D. (2007) *Sociology of Health and Healthcare*, 4th edn. Oxford: Blackwell Publishing.

Especially Chapter 4, Ethnicity and Health.

Useful websites

The National Childbirth Trust **www.nct.org.uk**
UK-based charity supporting new parents and parents-to-be.

Office for National Statistics **www.ons.gov.uk**
You can find census results and other statistics on this government site.

Chapter 5
Sexual and reproductive health in childbearing

Heather Passmore

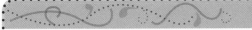

NMC Essential Skills Clusters

This chapter will address the following ESCs:

Cluster: Communication

3. Enable women to make choices about their care by informing women of the choices available to them and providing evidence-based information about benefits and risks of options so that women can make a fully informed decision.

*   Uses appropriate strategies to encourage and promote choice for all women.
*   Provides accurate, truthful and balanced information that is presented in such a way as to make it easily understood.
*   Discusses with women local/national information to assist with making choices, including local and national voluntary agencies and websites.

Cluster: Medical products management

1. Within the parameters of normal childbirth, ensure safe and effective practice through comprehensive knowledge of medicinal products, their actions, risks and benefits including the ability to recognise and respond safely to adverse drug events.

*   Uses knowledge and understanding of commonly supplied or administered medicinal products to the woman or baby in order to act promptly in cases where side effects and adverse reactions occur.

Chapter aims

After reading this chapter you will be able to:

*   promote holistic sexual healthcare for pregnant women;
*   provide sound contraceptive advice to childbearing women;
*   identify, signpost and appropriately refer women to other healthcare professions for screening, diagnosis and treatment of sexually transmitted infections and contraceptive issues;
*   reflect on factors that influence women's choices around sexual health and control of fertility.

Introduction

This chapter will consider anatomy and physiology related to reproductive health and sexual health, and models to promote discussion of the topic with women. Midwives' responsibilities to recognise the possibility of sexually transmitted infection (STI) and refer for investigation and treatment together with knowledge of contraceptive methods suitable for recently delivered women will be explored.

Anatomy and physiology

The biology of the vagina and its functions can make women susceptible to infection. The lining of the vagina is in folds (rugae) to facilitate coitus and passage of the fetus; it allows menstrual flow, supports the uterus and helps prevent ascending infection. Lactobacilli are the dominant bacteria in the healthy vagina resulting in a pH between 3.5–4.5. If the pH of the vagina becomes more alkaline (between 4.5–6.0) the growth of anaerobic bacteria is favoured, which may cause bacterial vaginosis. A discharge from the vaginal is normal, caused by cervical secretions and transudate from the blood vessels beneath the vaginal mucosa. In response to raised circulating oestrogen and progesterone in pregnancy, this discharge may increase in volume but should remain non-irritant and non-offensive. An offensive or irritating discharge is likely to be a symptom of an infection (see Table 5.1).

	Physiological	**Bacterial vaginosis**	**Candida albicans**	**Trichomonas vaginalis**
Detection	Increases in pregnancy/some hormonal contraceptive methods	50% Asymptomatic	10–20% Asymptomatic	10–50% Asymptomatic
Appearance	Clear/white	Thin/white grey	Thick/white	Thin/frothy
Smell	Odourless	Fishy (noted particularly after sex)	Not offensive	Offensive
Signs and Symptoms	None unless excessive	Usually nothing, may be some burning on micturition	Itchy/sore Vulval oedema and/or fissures	Itchy/sore Dysuria

Table 5.1: Comparison of characteristics of vaginal discharge

Providing sexual healthcare: the midwife's role

Sexual and reproductive health has been recognised as an area for midwifery public health intervention throughout the maternity pathway (DH, 2009). Midwives can contribute to maximising wellbeing and improve health in women and babies, as well as providing sound family planning advice (Directive 2005/36.EC of the European Parliament and of the Council). Midwives need to be knowledgeable about all contraceptive methods, their advantages, disadvantages, risks and benefits so they can help women choose an appropriate method and instruct them in its use. The majority of women, even those who have conceived through in vitro fertilisation, will have had sex without a condom in their attempt to become pregnant and therefore are at risk of transmission of sexually transmitted infections. Correlation of the highest rates of sexually transmitted infections to women aged 16–44 years and in particular those under 25, indicates midwives need to be aware of the significant effect of some infections on pregnancy, the neonate and the health of women (Public Health England [PHE], 2014). Opportunities to promote safe reproductive sexual health, with choice of effective contraception for optimum pregnancy spacing will contribute to worldwide reduction in maternal and infant mortality.

Good sexual and reproductive health is important to both individuals and society. Concepts of good sexual health acknowledge that it encompasses a range of feelings, abilities and activities, and means different things to different people at different ages. Respect for needs and views of others and the different nature of others enables individuals to feel happy and supported in a sexual identity. It provides correct information on fertility, contraception, STIs and ability to use information in personal decision-making and access to appropriate services for contraception, screening and treatment of infections.

Many different factors can influence relationships and safer sex, including:

- personal attitudes and beliefs;
- social norms;
- peer pressure;
- religious beliefs;
- culture;
- confidence and self-esteem;
- misuse of drugs and alcohol;
- coercion and abuse.

(DH, 2013b)

Many women remain sexually active during pregnancy, usually without barrier protection against sexually transmitted infections. However, pregnancy provides opportunities for screening for a variety of sexually transmitted infections such as syphilis, HIV, hepatitis B and in the under-25-year-olds, chlamydia, alongside other routine screening (NICE, 2008). The postnatal period is a time of physiological, psychological and social readjustment that can influence sexual and reproductive health. Women are usually receptive to health promotion during pregnancy, and contraceptive advice can be provided in the third trimester and during the postnatal period.

Activity 5.1   *Research and evidence-based practice*

Review the physiology of menstruation and spermatogenesis and changes in the vagina during pregnancy by selecting an appropriate anatomy and physiology book (for example Coad and Dunstall, 2012 or Stables and Rankin, 2010), then answer the following questions:

(a) What causes the anterior pituitary gland to increase production of follicle stimulating hormone?

(b) What does luteinising hormone do?

continued . . .

continued . . .

    (c)   What physiological sign may a woman detect to know that ovulation has occurred?

    (d)   What does the corpus luteum produce and what happens to this if fertilisation of an ovum does not occur?

    (e)   What is the lifespan of spermatozoa?

    (f)   During pregnancy how can vaginal discharge alter and why?

An outline answer to this activity is given at the end of the chapter.

Strategies for promoting sexual health

In 2001 the government published its first national strategy for sexual health and HIV (DH, 2001). Its aims were to:

- reduce transmission of HIV and STIs;
- reduce prevalence of undiagnosed HIV and STIs;
- lower unintended pregnancy rates;
- eradicate the stigma associated with HIV and STIs;
- improve health and social care for people living with HIV.

The Framework for Sexual Health Improvement in England (DH, 2013b) reaffirms many of these aims proposing that unwanted pregnancies will be reduced by ensuring people have access to the full range of contraception, and can actively plan how many children they want, and the spacing between pregnancies. The consequences of poor sexual health can be reduced through accurate, high quality and timely information that helps people make informed decisions about relationships, sex and sexual health. Midwives can contribute to this agenda (DH, 2013b).

Research summary: Sexual attitudes and practices

The third National Survey of Sexual Attitudes and Lifestyles on 15,162 men and women aged between 16–74 years resident in Britain (Mercer *et al.*, 2013) reported the following changes since 2001:

- women engaging in more sexual repertoires within heterosexual relationships, particularly oral and anal sex;
- greater acceptance of same sex relationships.

Attendance at sexual health clinics has increased over the last ten years with an increase in testing, concordant with recommended testing for HIV and syphilis in asymptomatic individuals (Sonnenberg *et al.*, 2013).

Unplanned pregnancy can have a negative effect on women's lives, resulting in poorer outcomes for both mother and baby and is a key public health issue. Increasing intervals between first sexual intercourse, cohabitation and childbearing means that the average woman in Britain will spend at least 30 years of her life avoiding pregnancy. Midwives have a role to play in achieving this (Wellings *et al.*, 2013).

Activity 5.2   *Critical thinking*

Write a definition of what sexual health means to you.

A concise definition of sexual health offered by Greenhouse (1995) is:

Enjoyment of sexual activity of one's choice, without causing or suffering physical or mental harm.

Other definitions are offered at the end of the chapter.

Painter and Adams (2004) provide a visual representation of sexual health in the form of a flower. They describe the roots as the political influences at macro level on sexual health while the stems relate to individuals' social and community experiences which can determine the strength to support the flower. The petals detail the many facets of sexual health that can aid awareness, which can be considered as contributing to good sexual health and also sexuality.

Taking a sexual health history

Midwives have considerable experience in taking a booking history from women that retrieves a significant amount of information, much of which is of a personal and sensitive nature. There are similarities to some of the requirements for taking a sexual health history (SSHA, 2004): a non-judgemental attitude; the ability to develop an effective practitioner–patient relationship; an awareness of the complexities of human relationships. However the ability to discuss matters of a sexual nature in a frank and open manner may be challenging to some midwives who may question whether it is necessarily part of their role, preferring to recommend women to specialist services.

Communication and sexual health

Robinson (1996, p420) maintains that sexual advice to childbearing women is 'often poorly given, inexact, inexplicit, euphemistic and misleading, allowing no opportunity for clarification and discussion of alternatives.' Robinson identifies three inter-related aspects that impact on sexual health and proposes a 'SEX' model to enable practitioners to utilise three domains of learning to explore knowledge and provide explanation and teaching on skills and attitudes with individuals.

- **Skills** (Psychomotor)
- **Emotions** (Affective)
- e**X**planation (Cognitive)

Examples of use of the 'SEX' model by a midwife are:

Sexuality

- **Skills** – communication, teach pelvic floor exercises, bladder control.
- **Emotion** – perineal pain, antenatal and labour debriefing, support in labour.
- e**X**planation – Antenatal: intercourse – safety, positions; Postnatal – when to resume, hormonal effects if breastfeeding.

Screening

- **Skills** – know when and how to screen with appropriate testing equipment.
- **Emotion** – develop a positive attitude, deal with anxiety from previous referral/detection of infection or doubts about sexuality.
- e**X**planation – Chlamydia screening for under-25-year-olds, postnatal screening for discharging eyes in the neonate cervical screening programme, breast awareness, risks.

Sexually transmitted infections

- **Skills** – know how to minimise risk, safer sex.
- **Emotion** – non-judgemental, destigmatise service provision.
- e**X**planation – risks of infection to mother and baby (+partner[s]), education re availability and access to screening (Robinson, 1996).

Sex during pregnancy

Neither midwives nor mothers may wish to readily discuss the topic of sex in pregnancy, perhaps due to embarrassment, or fear of being judged. Unless the woman is bleeding, has a placenta praevia or is experiencing pain, there is no reason why sexual activity should not continue. However in the first trimester fatigue, nausea or vomiting may reduce libido. Midwives can help to normalise the issue of sex in pregnancy by broaching the subject in a friendly, relaxed way, for example:

People often ask me whether it is OK to have sex . . .

In case you are wondering, your love life can carry on until . . .

and then pause to see if this elicits any response or questions from the mother (Quilliam, 2010).

Situation	Explanation
Positions best for sex during pregnancy	Woman on top, rear entry and side to side are usually the best for comfort and accessibility. Avoidance of deep and weight-bearing positions Avoid the woman being on her back to prevent dizziness caused by central venous compression
Use of various forms of stimulation	Most forms of stimulation including intercourse are safe
To start labour when woman overdue	Stimulation of cervix releases prostaglandins; also contained within seminal fluid and may stimulate uterine activity
Use of sex toys	As long as they are clean and used gently
Medical reason, e.g. placenta praevia, high blood pressure	Explain why and state a time limit if possible when sex is inadvisable
Either partner has a STI	Use protection to reduce transmission (avoid sex for at least 7 days after treatment)
Sex hurts or causes bleeding, discharge or cramps	Seek the advice of a midwife or obstetrician for an explanation

Table 5.2: Sex in pregnancy – giving information

Annon (1976) uses the PLISSIT model for the management of sexual problems:

P – Permission giving.

LI – Limited information.

SS – Specific suggestions.

IT – Intensive therapy.

Within a midwife's scope of practice (NMC, 2008) the midwife can facilitate the first step to give permission in order to elicit information and offer limited advice; however if there is any suggestion of abnormality in discharge or symptoms that may be associated with a sexually transmitted infection, a referral to a specialist genitourinary medicine (GUM) clinic would be required. The British Association for Sexual Health and HIV (BASHH – **www.bashh.org.uk**) provides online, regularly updated clinical guidance on sexually transmitted infections.

<table>
<tr><td>

Activity 5.3

</td><td>

Critical thinking

</td></tr>
</table>

Consider the statements below and refer back to Table 5.1 to guide you in communicating with women presenting with these sexual health needs:

(a) How will you ask a woman at routine antenatal visits about personal matters such as the nature of vaginal discharge?

(b) How do you ask a woman if she has changed her sexual partner or had other sexual partners during pregnancy? What advice would you give this woman?

(c) A 26-year-old married woman complains of vaginal soreness and itching at her 28-week visit. She has experienced this before, but it is much worse this time. You suggest she could access her local sexual health clinic for more specialist advice and screening but she appears reluctant to do so. What may be the reasons for this?

There are no specific answers to these questions.

Sexually transmitted infections

The prevalence of many sexually transmitted infections has risen in the UK (PHE, 2014). For more detailed information, review the relevant infection at: **http://www.bashh.org/BASHH/ Guidelines/Guidelines.aspx**

The most important behaviour a midwife can adopt is to raise awareness and facilitate discussion on concerns that a woman may have in relation to her risk of having a sexually transmitted infection. This necessitates the midwife to ask questions that relate to their sexual history including the nature of vaginal discharge and any change in sexual partner(s). If a woman presents with any symptoms suggestive of an infection referral to a specialist sexual health clinic (GUM) for full screening together with her partner(s) is strongly recommended. Referral for asymptomatic screening is recommended for women who change their sexual partner during pregnancy. Any woman (and her partner) requiring treatment for a sexually transmitted infection should be advised not to have vaginal, anal or oral sex and avoid any kind of skin contact with their partner until seven days have elapsed since both partners stopped treatment.

Human immunodeficiency virus (HIV)

HIV is a retrovirus which infects the immune system's cells, particularly the CD4 lymphocytes. It is present in an infected person's blood and other body fluids such as vaginal or rectal secretions, semen and breast milk. During the 'window' period, antibodies to HIV typically appear within 4–6 weeks after infection, but may take as long as 12 weeks. A flu-like illness, which may range from mild to significant, is experienced by 60% of people at this stage. Following seroconversion, the aysmptomatic stage of the infection starts which offers some explanation for the estimated 30% of undiagnosed cases (Baggaley, 2008). Two diagnostic markers, assessed via a blood test, are used to monitor HIV (see Coad and Dunstall, 2012, Chapter 10 for more information on immunology). The CD4 lymphocyte, a form of the T lymphocyte called the helper T cell, indicates the degree of immunosuppression and in non-infected individuals is usually >500 cells/mm^3 but can be variable. As the CD4 level falls (below 200 cells/mm^3) the patient is at risk of HIV-related opportunistic infections and tumours. The other diagnostic marker is the viral load which can range from undetectable to over a million copies/mL. The degree of viral replication is linked to the decline in CD4 count and disease progression. Antiretroviral therapy (ART), using a combination of different types of inhibitors, is used to reduce the viral load to undetectable levels. Management of ART is outside the scope of midwifery practice (NMC, 2008), however the midwife should encourage compliance with complex medication regimes and engagement with the multidisciplinary team who manage HIV.

The midwife should be competent to explain the risk of HIV transmission from mother and baby and offer appropriate information and support should a woman wish to opt out of routine screening for HIV. In the UK and Ireland antenatal HIV screening is routinely offered to all women, with a high uptake (>95% overall in England). HIV women are increasingly likely to be aware of their diagnosis pre-conceptually and in 2009, 39% of pregnancies in diagnosed women were a second or subsequent pregnancy following HIV diagnosis (Byrne *et al.*, 2013).

The National Study of HIV in Pregnancy and Childhood (NSHPC) is the confidential national (UK and Ireland) active reporting scheme for pregnancies in HIV-positive women, babies born to HIV positive women and other children with HIV infection (**www.ucl.ac.uk/nshpc**). A surveillance programme is maintained to evaluate antenatal HIV testing and mother to child transmission. Townsend *et al.* (2014) reports a four-fold drop in transmissions based on almost 12,500 pregnancies in diagnosed women having babies between 2000 to 2011, from 2.1% in 2000/2001 to 0.46% in 2010/11. Other reported changes are an increase in vaginal delivery among HIV positive women, though considerable maternity unit variation exists on this practice (Peters, 2014). A normal vaginal delivery is possible if a VL <50 copies/mL is achieved by 36 weeks (BHIVA, 2012).

Exclusive formula feeding should still be recommended to all HIV-positive mothers in the UK. Infant formula in the UK is affordable, feasible, acceptable, sustainable and safe, so complete avoidance of breastfeeding avoids any risk of transmission. Breastfeeding by women with detectable viraemia remains a safeguarding concern. However, women with fully suppressed HIV on ART, who choose to breastfeed against medical advice, should be supported to maximise adherence to maintain an undetectable HIV viral load throughout breastfeeding (BHIVA, 2014).

The diagnosis of any STI in pregnancy, but particularly HIV, can be devastating and the information given to mothers and their partners needs to be communicated sensitively, with dignity and compassion. Care in pregnancy will require midwives to work with others in genitourinary medical care and the specialist HIV team. Midwives can contribute to the prevention of STI by offering and referring women for screening during pregnancy and being aware of local sexual health service provision, availability and accessibility. Women should be encouraged to consistently and correctly use condoms until all sexual partners have had a sexual health screen.

Contraceptive care

Midwives are required to provide sound family planning advice and therefore need to know when fertility returns.

- For non-breastfeeding women, the earliest date of ovulation is day 28, with menstruation returning by week 6 (Glasier *et al.*, 1988).

- Ovulation is likely to be suppressed in breastfeeding women, returning when the frequency and duration of suckling decreases. Menstruation occurs on average 28.4 (range, 15–48) weeks after delivery for women who are breastfeeding. The mean time to initiation of ovulation is 33.6 (range, 14–51) weeks.

- The first 'true period' is defined as any bleeding lasting at least 2 days, requiring the use of sanitary protection for at least 1 day, followed by a second bleeding episode within the next 21–70 days.

- Menstruation may be regarded as the return of fertility; some women may ovulate and therefore conceive if contraception has not been started prior to menstruation.

- Inter-pregnancy intervals of less than 6 months are associated with an increased risk of negative perinatal outcome (Smith *et al.*, 2003) and can pose increased risk to maternal health (Conde-Agudelo *et al.*, 2006).

Resumption of sexual activity

The weeks following childbirth can be a time of significant change for women. Sex can be influenced by bio/psycho/social concerns, for example lower circulating oestrogen levels, while breastfeeding may cause vaginal dryness; orgasm may cause an oxytocin rise and stimulate milk leakage; fear of dyspareunia (painful sex), pain from perineal or abdominal wounds and concern that they will be interrupted by the baby crying.

The midwife needs to convey information regarding resumption of sexual activity following birth with sensitivity, and women should be reassured that it is a very individual matter. For some couples this may not be for some months; a small proportion have still not resumed sexual intercourse after 6 months (Barrett *et al.*, 2000). A systematic review of six articles suggests a possible association between sexual dysfunction and assisted vaginal delivery (Hicks *et al.*, 2004), however, this is disputed by von Brummen *et al.* (2006).

Sexual activity may be resumed when both partners feel ready (FSRH, 2009). However, following a few deaths from air embolism following sexual intercourse, the Centre for Maternal and Child Enquiries(CMACE, 2011) advises recommending abstinence for 6 weeks, or gentle intercourse avoiding positions (e.g. all fours) that might allow excess air to be forced into the vagina (CMACE, 2011, p156).

Sexual activity after childbirth

Women and their partners may be reassured by the following information:

- The time to resume sexual activity will vary between couples.
- There is no set time frame in which sexual activity should have resumed.
- Both partners need to be physically and emotionally ready.
- Some people may experience difficulties with sexual activity following the birth of their child.
- Sexual desire or sex drive may be low in the first few months.
- Any difficulties or concerns should be discussed with a health professional.

(FSRH, 2009)

Glasier (1996) suggests that contraceptive advice may be best offered in the antenatal period and the 36-week visit would be an ideal time, providing women with the opportunity to consider and investigate the options prior to the birth of her baby. However NICE (2006b) continues to recommend that advice about contraceptive methods and their use should be discussed within the first week following delivery.

There are no reports of ovulation prior to 28 days following delivery (FSRH, 2009), therefore, allowing for the potential seven-day survival of sperm, contraception should be used from day 21 following delivery. The midwife should be knowledgeable about all forms of contraception to enable the woman and her partner to choose a method that suits their individual requirements. The personal and family medical history of the woman is required, which should be combined with information on method effectiveness and likely user compliance.

Contraceptive decision-making can be complex and women may base their decisions on personal beliefs and reported concerns over side effects and risks rather than systematically weighing up the pros and cons of a method determined by safety, efficacy, ease of use, availability and accessibility. A midwife must have a good knowledge of all contraceptive methods to fulfil the EC directive to be able 'to provide sound family planning advice'. In addition the ability to take a good personal and family medical history, plus sexual and reproductive history, will elicit any of the contraindications to any method and this information can be supported by referral to the UK Medical Eligibility Guidelines (RCOG, 2009a). A midwife should be able to give verbal and written or online access to information on mode and duration of action, failure rate, side effects and risks, the benefits of the methods and when to seek advice, together with advise on safer sex.

Knowledge on the types of contraception that can be offered to women can be found on the following website. Please make sure you access it: **www.fpa.org.uk/help-and-advice/ contraception-help**

Evidence-based guidance can be found at: **http//www.fsrh.org/pages/clinical_guidance.asp**

The effectiveness of a contraceptive method is calculated using the Pearl Index, which indicates the number of failures of a method per 100,000 women years of use (Trussell and Portman, 2013). The Family Planning Association converts this figure to a more positive expression of percentage effectiveness, which is used in their leaflets on contraceptive methods, and allows women and their partners easier comparison between methods. However the effectiveness has two components: the method effectiveness, which is derived from perfect use; and the user effectiveness, as patterns of use are not always compliant with manufacturer's/practitioner's instructions, derived from typical use (see Table 5.3). This was one of the reasons NICE (2005) recommend the use of long-acting reversible contraception to aid concordance and reduce unwanted conception, as well as cost-effectiveness. Women who are fully informed and able to choose their method of contraception are likely to achieve greater method compliance.

No user failure	User failure
These do not depend on the woman remembering to take or use contraception	*These depend upon the woman remembering to use or think about regularly or each time sex occurs. Effectiveness is affected by compliance with instructions for use.*
Contraceptive injection >99%	Contraceptive patch >99%
Implant >99%	Combined pill >99%
Intrauterine system (IUS) >99%	Progestogen-only pill 99%
Intrauterine device (IUD) >99%	Male condom 98% – best use
Female sterilisation 1 in 200	Female condom 95%
Male sterilisation 1 in 2000	Diaphragm/cap with spermicide 92–96%
	Natural family planning >98% with multiple index methods
	Lactational amenorrhoea 98%

Table 5.3: Method compliance classification and effectiveness rates

Guillebaud and MacGregor (2013) describe a dilemma in contraceptive usage between increasing effectiveness that tends to be associated with increased health risks, whereas the methods with lower effectiveness have better safety profiles. A midwife should therefore have up-to-date knowledge (NMC, 2015) on the risks and benefits of various contraceptives methods as well as the method effectiveness.

Advice on contraception

Activity 5.4   *Critical thinking*

Use a PESTLE analysis as a framework to consider the macro factors that can affect contraceptive usage, under each of the following headings.

Factors affecting contraceptive use:

- **P**olitical
- **E**conomic
- **S**ocial
- **T**echnological
- **L**egal
- **E**nvironmental/**E**ducational

Discuss your PESTLE analysis with a peer and list your characteristics for the 'ideal contraceptive'.

Some suggestions are given at the end of the chapter.

Factors influencing contraceptive use

A consideration of the factors that influence contraceptive use together with the features of an ideal contraceptive reveals the problem that sexually active people encounter in deciding upon, obtaining and using contraception. The midwife should utilise verbal communication to provide evidence-based information in a form that is understood by a woman and her partner. Information should be in accordance with cultural practices and provided in a form that is accessible to women and their partners, taking account of any specific additional needs (NICE, 2006b). Women and their families can be advised to access information on each of the contraceptive methods via the Family Planning Association website, which also has a 'My Contraceptive Tool' to support decision-making (FPA, no date).

UK Medical Eligibility Criteria

The UK Medical Eligibility Criteria (UKMEC) provides a summary for practitioners for all common reversible methods of contraception indicating a category for use. This is derived from World Health Organization criteria that have been adapted for UK use and is continually reviewed. It provides a score that easily indicates to a practitioner the suitability of use as per Table 5.4 below.

UK category	Hormonal contraception, intrauterine devices and barrier method
1	A condition for which there is **no restriction for the use** of the contraceptive method
2	A condition where the **advantages of using the method generally outweigh the theoretical or proven risks**
3	A condition where the **theoretical or proven risks usually outweigh the advantages of using the method**
4	A condition, which represents an **unacceptable health risk** if the contraceptive is used
NB	For certain conditions the category may change depending on whether the method is to be initiated [I] or continued [C].

Table 5.4: UK Medical Eligibility Criteria for use of contraceptive methods

Ref: Faculty of Sexual and Reproductive Healthcare (2009).

For example, the guidance for contraception for postnatal women from the Faculty of Sexual and Reproductive Health indicates a UKMEC eligibility criterion of 2 for combined hormonal contraception (COC) if the woman had hypertension or cholestasis in pregnancy, while any intrauterine device is classed as category 4 if the woman has gestational trophoblastic neoplasia (hydatidiform mole, invasive mole, placental tumour) with persistently elevated β-hCG levels.

Knowledge of the physiological changes in coagulation during pregnancy and the associated risks of venous thromboembolism (VTE) in pregnancy can be utilised by midwives to explain the risks of this condition and contraception for women using the guidance below:

- Risk of VTE in women of reproductive age 4–5/10,000 women.
- Risk of VTE in COC is approximately twice that of new users:
  - risk highest in first few months;
  - risk returns to that of non-users within weeks;
  - restarting after 4-week break increases risk.
- Pregnancy risk of VTE 29/10,000 women.
- Post-partum risk of VTE is 300–400/10,000 women.

For this reason COC would not be started until day 21 following delivery to avoid increasing the VTE risk (UKMEC <21 days = 3).

Long-acting reversible contraception	Short-acting hormonal reversible contraception	Spontaneous reversible contraception
Implant (Nexplanon)	Combined pill (COC)	Condoms – male/female
Copper coils (IUD)	Contraceptive patch/ vaginal ring	Diaphragms and caps
Hormone coil Mirena/Jaydess – (IUS)	Progestogen only pill – (Desogestrel 75 mg)	Natural family planning, including lactational amenorrhoea
Injectables (e.g Depo-Provera 150 mg IM; Sayana Press® 104 mg SC)	Progestogen only pills (POP – levenorgestrel or norithesterone in various doses)	Withdrawal

Table 5.5: Classification of reversible contraceptive methods
NB: Spontaneous does not necessarily mean unplanned.

Emergency contraception

If women have unprotected sexual intercourse (UPSI), after day 21 they should be advised to access emergency contraception and the midwife should be aware of how to access the local service and direct the woman accordingly.

There are three types available, presented in order of effectiveness.

- Insertion of a copper intrauterine device (98% effective), can be fitted after day 28 without restriction. It can be fitted in the first 120 hours following first UPSI in a cycle or within five days from the earliest estimated date of ovulation and could be retained as long-term contraception.

- Ulipristal acetate 30 mg (ellaOne® [POM]), a progestogen only method, can be given orally as a single dose within 120 hours of UPSI or contraceptive failure to delay ovulation (FSRH, 2011). It affects breast milk, which should be discarded for 7 days.

- Levonorgestrel 1.5 mg (Levonelle 1500 [POM]), a progestogen only method, can be administered once orally within 72 hours of UPSI (possibly up to 96 hours), to delay ovulation (84% effective).

Alternatively in breastfeeding women the benefits and risks of emergency contraception should be considered in the context of the woman's low risk of pregnancy if fully breastfeeding, the disadvantages of stopping breastfeeding for one week after Ulipristal, and the availability/ acceptability of other methods (FSRH, 2013).

Pre-conceptual care for future pregnancies

Women should be encouraged to plan for future pregnancies to ensure they are in the best possible health for conception. They should be advised to:

- have a sexual health check, particularly if there has been a change of partner in the last year;
- discontinue hormonal contraception 3 months prior to planned conception;
- start folic acid and vitamin D supplementation;
- check rubella antibody status;
- aim to have a BMI within the 20–25 range;
- stop smoking and review any other substance misuse;
- consult with their general practitioner to review the management and medications for pre-existing medical conditions.

(Passmore and Chenery-Morris, 2013)

Special considerations

Dyspareunia (painful sex)

The relationship between the mother and a midwife can facilitate a discussion on whether sexual activity is painful, if it has been resumed prior to handover of care to a health visitor. This question can be asked between 2–6 weeks after birth. If dyspareunia is experienced and the woman suffered perineal trauma at birth, assessment of the perineum should be offered (NICE, 2006b). A water-based lubricant gel to help ease discomfort during intercourse may be advised, particularly if a woman is breastfeeding. If a woman expresses anxiety about resuming intercourse, reasons for this should be explored and if this continues the woman should be advised to seek medical evaluation (NICE, 2006b).

Women with same sex partners

The midwife should be sensitive to offering contraceptive advice if it is deemed completely unnecessary by a woman as she may be in a same sex relationship. If a homosexual female has had previous male partners or shares sex toys, it is advisable for these women to remain within the cervical screening programme and access STI screening (Fish, 2009).

Cervical cytology screening and pregnancy

In women under 25 years old cervical cancer is very rare, but prevalence of human papilloma virus is high: one in six smears are abnormal. However, all women over 25 should be encouraged to access cervical screening irrespective of whether they received an HPV vaccination as a teenager.

Activity 5.5   *Research and evidence-based practice*

Read the NHS National Screening Programmes, Cervical Screening: The Facts of Health leaflet (**www.cancerscreening.nhs.uk/cervical/publications/the-facts-other-languages.html**) and answer the following questions.

(a)   What is:

- the purpose of cervical screening and its limitations?

- the likelihood of a normal test result?

- the meaning of a normal test result?

- the meaning of being recalled following an abnormal test result?

(b)   What advice would you give in booking a 29-year-old woman who has not attended a routine recall for cervical screening, as her first test was normal?

A suggested answer is given at the end of the chapter.

Women called for a recall smear following abnormal result should attend for a smear in the second trimester. The receipt of abnormal cervical smear results in pregnancy will undoubtedly cause anxiety for the woman requiring additional support from the midwife. The primary aim of colposcopy for pregnant women is to exclude invasive disease and to defer biopsy or treatment until the woman has delivered. Cone, wedge and diathermy loop biopsies are all associated with a risk of haemorrhage. The incidence of invasive cervical cancer in pregnancy is low and pregnancy itself does not have an adverse effect on the prognosis (NHSCSP, 2010).

Sexual abuse and trafficking of women (see also Chapter 7 on Domestic abuse)

Midwives should be alert and sensitive to women who may report that they have been sexually assaulted in pregnancy, as this may require referral to a variety of agencies including safeguarding, social care and the police. They may visit the local Sexual Assault Referral Centre for investigations including screening for infection, DNA analysis and access to support.

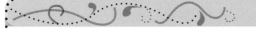 **Chapter summary**

This chapter has examined the components of sexual health and considered models that may assist midwives to communicate with mothers and their families on these personal, sensitive and often private issues. To fulfil a fundamental role of the midwife it is vital that midwives feel confident in their knowledge and how to keep this updated, in order to provide contemporary advice on contraception and sexual health appropriate

continued . . .

continued . . .

to a woman's individual needs with appropriate referral to specialist services. Midwives develop a continued relationship with women during pregnancy and the puerperium, providing opportunities to discuss intimate concerns and revisit them. This public health role enables midwives to make an important contribution to the promotion of both maternal and infant health by prevention of, recognition and referral for early treatment of sexually transmitted infections and avoidance of unplanned pregnancy through the effective use of contraception.

Activities: brief outline answers

Activity 5.1 Research and evidence-based practice [page 79]

Before ovulation	After ovulation
Follicle stimulating hormone (FSH) produced from anterior pituitary in response to low oestrogen levels. (negative feedback) prepares the 'dominant follicle' in the ovary	Following ovulation the follicle shrinks to become the corpus luteum.
The ovarian follicle increases and produces oestrogen. Increasing oestrogen levels are required to produce a positive feedback mechanism, which causes a surge in both FSH and luteinising hormone (LH) levels.	The corpus luteum produces oestrogen and progesterone which prepare the lining of the uterus to receive a fertilised ovum for implantation.
The LH surge causes the ovarian follicle to rupture, ovulation, which is usually followed by a rise in basal body temperature of between 0.2–0.5°C. Ovulation is of variable length in the cycle. The life span of an oocyte is a maximum of 24 hours.	If fertilisation does not occur then progesterone and oestrogen levels decline and menstruation occurs. Ovulation to menstruation constant length – 14 days.

Male reproductive physiology:

- Sperm are produced at the rate of 1000 per second from each testicle.
- Semen contains about 80 million sperm per mL.
- About 3 mL of semen are released with each ejaculation.
- About 240 million sperm per ejaculation.
- Only one sperm enters the ovum at fertilisation.
- The lifespan of sperm is 5–7 days.

Activity 5.2 Critical thinking [page 81]

Your definition of sexual health may include aspects of the following Department of Health definition:

> *Sexual health is an important part of physical and mental health. It is a key part of our identity as human beings together with fundamental human rights to privacy, a family life and living free from discrimination. Essential elements of good sexual health are equitable relationships, sexual fulfilment with access to information and services to avoid the risk of unintended pregnancy, illness or disease.*

(DH, 2001)

Definition of the World Health Organization:

> *Sexual health is a state of physical, emotional, mental and social wellbeing in relation to sexuality; it is not merely the absence of disease, dysfunction or infirmity. Sexual health requires a positive and respectful approach to sexuality and sexual relationships, as well as the possibility of having pleasurable and safe sexual experiences, free of coercion, discrimination and violence. For sexual health to be attained and maintained, the sexual rights of all persons must be respected, protected and fulfilled.*

(WHO, 2006)

However the WHO believes that sexual health cannot be defined, understood or made operational without a broad consideration of sexuality, which underlies important behaviours and outcomes related to sexual health. The working definition of sexuality is:

> *…a central aspect of being human throughout life encompasses sex, gender identities and roles, sexual orientation, eroticism, pleasure, intimacy and reproduction. Sexuality is experienced and expressed in thoughts, fantasies, desires, beliefs, attitudes, values, behaviours, practices, roles and relationships. While sexuality can include all of these dimensions, not all of them are always experienced or expressed. Sexuality is influenced by the interaction of biological, psychological, social, economic, political, cultural, legal, historical, religious and spiritual factors.*

(WHO, 2006)

Activity 5.4 Critical thinking [page 89]

Your PESTLE analysis of factors affecting contraceptive usage could have included:

- **Political** – total fertility rate, teenage pregnancy rate, abortion rate, rising STIs, sexual health is a target area for government policy.
- **Economic** – organisation and management, availability and access, costs and services, quality of care, dispensing budget, ring-fenced money to meet sexual health targets.
- **Social** – reproductive health status, users' perspectives, gender, family, friends, peers, religious/cultural normal, children (the need for sons), relationships.
- **Technological** – Method-mix, method characteristics, effectiveness, safety, internet and apps to direct users to services and provide reminders on method use.
- **Legal** – Abortion Law 1967, Human Fertilisation and Embryology Act 1990, Sexual Offences Act 2004, legal intercourse for intercourse, Fraser competency.
- **Environmental** – discharge of hormones into water courses, recyclable or filling landfill sites.
- **Educational** – social class, knowledge, career aspirations, self-esteem, beliefs, myths.

You might have found the ideal contraceptive to be:

- 100% reversible;
- 100% effective;
- 100% unforgettable;
- 100% convenient – not related to having sex;
- 100% free from side effects;
- 100% protective against STIs;
- possessing other non-contraceptive benefits;
- 100% maintenance free;
- acceptable to every culture, religion and political view;
- cheap and easily available;
- not dependent upon healthcare practitioners' to access.

(Adapted from Guillebaud and MacGregor, 2013)

Activity 5.5(b) Research and evidence-based practice [page 93]

- If a woman who has been called for routine screening is now pregnant – defer test until 3 months post-delivery.
- Unless a pregnant woman with a negative history has gone beyond three years without having cervical screening then the test should be postponed until 3 months post-delivery.
- If previous test abnormal, and now pregnant, the test should not be delayed but should be taken in mid-trimester unless there is a clinical contraindication.

Further reading

Coad, J. and Dunstall, M. (2012) *Anatomy and Physiology for Midwives*, 3rd edn. Edinburgh: Churchill Livingstone.
See especially Chapter 4: Reproductive Cycles.

DH (2013) *A Framework for Sexual Health Improvement in England (Best Practice Guidance).* London: Department of Health.

Glasier, A.F., Logan, J., McGrew, T.J. (1996) Who gives advice about postpartum contraception? *Contraception*, 53: 217–220.

Greenhouse, P. (1995) A definition of sexual health. *BMJ*, 310: 1468.

Guillebaud, J. and MacGregor, A. (2013) *Contraception: Your Questions Answered*, 6th edn. Edinburgh: Elsevier.

Robinson, J. (1996) The SEX model of sexual health. *British Journal of Midwifery*, 4 (8): 420–424.

Stables, D. and Rankin, J. (2010) *Physiology in Childbearing; with Anatomy and Related Biosciences*, 3rd edn. Edinburgh: Baillière Tindall Elsevier.
See especially Chapter 6: Fertility Control.

Useful websites

The British Association for Sexual Health and HIV (BASHH)

www.bashh.org.uk
Provides online, regularly updated clinical guidance on sexually transmitted infections.

The Faculty for Sexual and Reproductive Health

www.fsrh.org
Provides online, regularly updated clinical guidance on contraception.

Chapter 6
Perinatal mental health

Sam Chenery-Morris

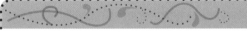

NMC Standards for Pre-registration Midwifery Education

This chapter will address the following competencies:

Domain: Effective midwifery practice

Provide seamless care, and where appropriate, interventions in partnership with women and other care providers during the antenatal period which:

- are appropriate for the woman's assessed needs, context and culture;
- promote their continuing health and wellbeing;
- are evidence-based;
- are consistent with the management of risk;
- draw upon the skills of others to optimise health outcomes and resource use.

Care for and monitor women during the puerperium, offering necessary evidence-based advice and support regarding the baby and self-care. This will include:

- Enabling women to address issues about their own, their babies' and their families' health and social wellbeing.
- Monitoring and supporting women who have postnatal depression or other mental illnesses.

NMC Essential Skills Clusters

This chapter will address the following ESCs:

Cluster: Communication

Women can trust/expect a newly registered midwife to:

7. Provide care that is delivered in a warm, sensitive and compassionate way.
8. Be confident in their own role and within a multidisciplinary/multi-agency team.

Cluster: Initial consultation between the woman and the midwife

2. Complete an initial consultation accurately ensuring women are at the centre of care.

Introduction

During your midwifery course so far you will have learned many new words. Terminology is important in midwifery because it makes ideas and events more specific if the correct word is used. In this chapter the term 'perinatal' will be used. A simple definition of the perinatal period is the time before and after birth. Thus perinatal is the period around or near the natal (birth) event. The use of the term perinatal, instead of antenatal or postnatal is preferred. This is because women can exhibit symptoms of mental illness across the time surrounding birth; they may not only fit into one period before birth, antenatal, or after birth, the postnatal period, but have symptoms that span these times. However, with that said, because maternity care is divided into episodes including pre-conceptual, antenatal, during birth or intrapartum and postnatal periods, this chapter will start with the role of the midwife and others pre-conceptually. It then covers the role of the midwife in the antenatal period, and considers screening and what the common mental illnesses are. There are few intrapartum considerations so this chapter will end with the postnatal period.

Mental disorders which occur during pregnancy and early motherhood, or 'perinatal mental illness', is a serious public and private health issue. The public health concerns regard depression and other forms of mental illness as a leading cause of poor maternal health and can lead to negative effects on the development of children. Privately the detrimental consequences of perinatal mental illness on the woman and her family can have long-lasting and devastating effects in their lives, including morbidity and mortality. There are many public policies to prevent, recognise and treat mental illness promptly and appropriately so the public and private effects are minimised.

To address the needs of women regarding their mental health assessment, this chapter continues the underlying theme of this book, that communication between you, the midwife, and the woman is paramount. The woman and her family should be at the centre of any discussions and decisions made.

The role of the midwife

The publications, national policies and guidelines which aim to support practitioners caring for pregnant women with perinatal mental illness and guide care include the National Institute for Health and Care Excellence's (NICE) *Antenatal and Postnatal Mental Health* (NICE, 2014c) and the *National Service Framework for Children, Young People and Maternity Services* (DH/DFeS, 2004). Key publications (NICE, 2008; Draycott *et al.*, 2011; NICE, 2014b; 2014c) all recommend that at a woman's first contact with services, in both the antenatal and postnatal periods, that healthcare professionals, often the midwife, should ask questions to identify mental health issues.

The latest guidance (NICE, 2014c) is more explicit about pre-conceptual counselling for women with existing or previous mental health problems than before. It states women with severe previous or past mental health problems should be referred to specialist mental health services for counselling. The counselling will advise them on their risks according to the type of disorder they have or had and its treatment options in pregnancy. Women on psychotropic drugs need particular advice about their treatment (see NICE, 2014c, p19 for more on this). As a midwife you are unlikely to be involved with women pre-conceptually. So, this pre-conceptual referral will be implemented by GPs and practice nurses or other health professionals who see women of childbearing age with known previous or existing mental illness. However, in the antenatal period you, the midwife, will need to identify and refer those at risk of serious perinatal mental illness urgently to psychiatric services. To understand this, you need to know what serious perinatal mental illness is and what a psychiatric service is. This chapter will then consider the questions a midwife should ask to identify mental health issues.

There are three terms used in healthcare: primary, secondary and tertiary services. The primary care sector is usually the first point of contact with a health professional. The GP is often contacted first if a patient is unwell; in pregnancy it can be the midwife and following birth the health visitor. Primary care providers often co-ordinate other care options and make referrals to other services. Secondary care is the next line of care offered if more specialised input is required; the woman is usually referred for this extra care. It includes district general hospital outpatient clinics, to see a consultant or specialised community teams.

In midwifery, a midwife would see all pregnant women; in primary care, those with risk factors would be referred to and see a consultant, usually a consultant obstetrician. Sometimes the woman's pregnancy care continues under the direction of the consultant; for other women it is referred back to the midwife. Secondary care can also be provided by a referral from the obstetrician to a psychiatrist as an outpatient appointment. The obstetrician discusses and plans the pregnancy and birth plans when there are complications in conjunction with midwifery care. A psychiatrist would discuss and plan the woman's mental healthcare; this may be with an obstetrician and a midwife offering the pregnancy care. Tertiary care is highly specialised consultative care often provided for inpatients referred from primary or secondary services. It is this form of urgent specialised consultative care that women who have serious mental illness may require.

	Who?	**Supported by**	**Purpose**
Primary care	GP, midwife, health visitor	Voluntary and self-help agencies	Universal recognition and detection for all pregnant women
Secondary care	Outpatient clinics, consultant obstetricians and consultant psychiatrist clinics	Substance misuse services, community perinatal services, community psychiatric nurses (CPN)	Assessment of women with previous moderate or severe mental illness or present history of moderate illness
Tertiary care	Mother and baby unit inpatient care	Other professionals, midwife, health visitor, GP, community psychiatrist services	Women with severe current psychosis or depression

Table 6.1: Primary, secondary and tertiary care

Adapted from Royal College of Psychiatrists, 2008.

Now you understand the services offered we turn to the definitions of perinatal mental illness.

Perinatal psychiatric disorders

Definitions of mild, moderate and severe (as stated in Table 6.2) are frequently used to describe experiences of mental illness. To understand these definitions some types and specific diagnoses of these illnesses will be considered. Mild and moderate illness is usually managed in primary care, which means in the community under the direction of a GP, but referrals and treatments may be made with discussions with outpatient services and community specialists. Severe mental illness will require more specialist services.

Mild and moderate mental illness – treated often by GP (primary) and sometimes supported by community services (secondary)	**Severe mental illness – treated by specialist services and psychiatrists (tertiary care)**
Anxiety, panic attacks	Schizophrenia
Depression	Severe depression
Post-traumatic stress disorder	Bipolar disorder
Obsessive-compulsive disorders	Psychotic episodes

Table 6.2: Who treats mental illness?

The definitions of mild, moderate and severe may not be helpful to women since the woman experiencing mild anxiety may be feeling significant distress, but for healthcare professionals and midwives these classifications may help assess risk. The risk of relapse is higher in severe forms of mental illness, for instance the rate of relapse in the postnatal period is increased if a woman has bipolar disorder.

A perinatal psychiatric disorder is another term used in textbooks to refer to perinatal mental illness. The list of psychiatric disorders is, according to some, over 300 separate diagnoses (APA, 2013). You will see there are only a few offered in this chapter, namely, the most common ones. Psychiatric disorders span the lifetime, which means they can occur in childhood, adolescence, adulthood and older age; most start in childhood and adolescence (Paananen *et al.*, 2013). The causes of these can be varied. Genetics have a role; some families seem to have more incidences of psychiatric disorders than others, and thus taking a family history is one factor that can be used to identify a possible risk of mental illness. Traumatic birth or events in early childhood have also been attributed to psychiatric disorders or exposure to toxins during pregnancy. Mental disorders are linked to many family social risks such as family breakdown or early parental death, receipt of sustenance benefits and low educational attainment (Paananen *et al.*, 2013). Alternatively mental wellbeing is affected by life experiences, including stress, violence or abuse (Howard *et al.*, 2013).

Psychiatric disorders are common during pregnancy; they can occur for the first time, or a reoccurrence of a previous mental health disorder may manifest. The most common disorders during pregnancy are anxiety, depression, bipolar disorder, schizophrenia and postnatal psychotic disorders. The term postnatal depression should no longer be used because it is not specific enough to determine the exact nature of the disorder, or for the term to be meaningful to practitioners, due to its overuse (Raynor and England, 2010).

Activity 6.1   *Reflection*

With a fellow student, using Table 6.2 above or your own knowledge, list as many mental health terms and diagnoses as you can. Use a dictionary to define these terms. Consider whether your understanding of these terms was correct or limited.

There are no suggestions at the end of this chapter, but we hope the chapter will help clarify some of the terms you came up with.

Now you have considered some of the terms associated with recognising perinatal mental illness, we will consider detecting women at risk.

Assessing mental health

Over the years there have been a number of validated screening tools used to ask women about their mental health. You may have heard of the Edinburgh Postnatal Depression Screening (EPDS) tool, for instance. Nowadays, there is a shift away from screening women to predicting and detecting which individuals and which groups of women are more likely to develop perinatal mental illness. The EDPS is a questionnaire which asks a series of questions to all postnatal women. It was used as a screening tool for signs and symptoms of depression. The newer idea of assessing individuals comes from knowledge that certain factors are more likely to predict and can then be used to detect which women are at greater risk of mental illness, as opposed to looking for signs and symptoms once they have occurred.

Two short focused questions that address mood and interest are now recommended (NICE, 2014c). These two questions are as good at predicting ill health as many questions (Whooley *et al.*, 1997). Since time is limited in many healthcare interactions, and the antenatal booking interview between the midwife and women needs to establish a relationship, exchange information and assess risk, asking two questions is as reliable as undertaking the more time consuming multiple question screening tools.

The two questions are:

1. 'During the past month, have you often been bothered by feeling down, depressed or hopeless?'
2. 'During the past month, have you often been bothered by having little interest or pleasure in doing things?'

Each question requires a yes or no answer from women; however as a midwife you will also notice their body language, eye contact and consider how the woman replies as indicators of her mood and interest; these non-verbal responses may incline the midwife to ask further probing questions.

The Whooley questions have been developed (Arroll *et al.*, 2005) and a further 'help' question should be used if the woman answers yes to either of the initial questions:

3. 'Is this something you feel you need or want help with?'

This question has three possible answers: yes, no and not now. A positive reply for these answers indicates a referral to the GP is required (NICE, 2014c). If you think a woman's mental health is more severe than she is saying, a referral to specialist mental health services is recommended. It is hoped that you, as a student midwife having been out on placement, have seen midwives ask these questions in clinical practice, at antenatal booking appointments and postnatal visits. However, research of student midwives shows that how some midwives ask the sensitive questions is like a tick list and could be more woman-centred (Jarrett, 2014). Think about how you ask the questions and whether you are sensitive to the woman's answers.

In the latest antenatal and postnatal guidance (NICEc, 2014c) two further screening questions have been suggested. It may take a while for these to filter into everyday midwifery practice, but they have been introduced to help practitioners identify commonly misrecognised anxiety. The questions come from the General Anxiety Disorder scale item 7.

1. Over the last two weeks, have you been feeling nervous, anxious or on the edge?
2. Over the last two weeks, have you not been able to stop or control worrying?

These questions have a score attached to them: 0 for a response of not at all; 1 for on several days over the last two weeks; 2 for more than half the time; and 3 for nearly every day. If a woman says nearly every day, she needs to be referred to her GP, unless you feel she has other risk factors and specialist mental health services would be more appropriate – in which case refer her there, but remember to inform the GP as well.

The next method used by midwives to predict and detect women at risk of serious or moderate mental illness, in addition to the mood and interest questions, is to ask women if they have previous or present serious mental illness. If they have the midwife needs to ask whether they have had or are having treatment for this. Treatment may indicate the illness was more severe than they recognised or are willing to admit. Finally the woman's family history of mental illness is also enquired about; of particular note is a first degree relative (sister, mother or daughter) with severe mental illness. The reasons for these further questions help assess the risk for this woman for recurring mental illness and/or whether a change in her current treatment is required.

Treatment choices for moderate and severe mental illness include self-help approaches, counselling, cognitive behavioural therapy and other psychological treatments, which can be continued in pregnancy (Harvey *et al.*, 2012). Other treatment options include medications which may need to be reviewed or altered during the pregnancy. The umbrella term used for the drugs which alter chemical levels in the brain and affect mood and behaviour is psychotropic medications. The medications used fall into four categories: anxiolytics, antidepressants, antipsychotics and mood stabilisers. Anxiolytics are used to treat anxiety and can help induce sleep. These drugs can be addictive and are usually only prescribed for short periods. Antidepressants are prescribed for continued low mood and depression as well as eating disorders and obsessive-compulsive disorders. These drug treatments are frequently used for a period of six months or more and ceasing medication is usually a gradual process. Antipsychotics are used to treat psychotic conditions such as schizophrenia or manic phases of bipolar disorders. Mood stabilisers include lithium for treating bipolar disorders; however this drug can have toxic effects, so careful monitoring is essential. Lithium has been known to have a teratogenic effect of the developing fetus, which causes congenital abnormalities, and therefore women on this drug need counselling to ascertain the benefits of the treatment for their mental wellbeing and the side effects for their fetus. The next activity will help familiarise yourself with the medications used to treat mental illness.

Activity 6.2   *Research and evidence-based practice*

Access and read the NICE (2014c) antenatal and postnatal mental health guidance.

This document gives clear guidelines about which women should be referred and how urgently they require additional perinatal mental healthcare. It also states which medications are less risky during pregnancy and lactation. Use the BNF online or a search engine to help you further understand terminology used in the guidelines.

There are no suggested answers at the end of this chapter as you will look these medications up according to your pre-existing knowledge and interest.

This activity may be difficult, but accessing and reading key documents and then following up words in the document you do not understand helps improve your knowledge. Remember though, you are training to be a midwife, where the key responsibility is to identify women at risk and to refer as appropriate, not diagnose illness or prescribe treatments. Research shows qualified midwives and other practitioners sometimes have difficulties supporting women with perinatal mental illness (Schytt and Waldenström, 2013), so you are not alone if this chapter is initially hard to grasp. Collectively more can be done to support and treat these women; referral is the first step. As the woman's midwife and advocate, you will explain to the women you refer why they need extra support and to continue on their present medication until they are seen by a doctor. A different medication may be necessary, but this will be decided by the doctor in discussion with the woman and her symptoms. To help you further understand this guidance the following sections will help you with the terms and specific disorders you are likely to encounter.

The key message is to ask *all* women as early in the pregnancy as possible about their current and previous mental health. This is to determine which women may require more support and surveillance or treatment during this time. Remember though, a woman needs to feel comfortable if she is to answer the questions honestly (Brealey *et al.*, 2010). An Australian study (Rollans *et al.*, 2013) explored the content and process of an antenatal booking interview, looking especially at the way psychosocial aspects of the women's lives were assessed. It is the psychosocial, or psychological and social aspects of women's lives that are often factors which can be seen as risks for poor mental wellbeing or mental illness (we will come back to these shortly). In this study (Rollans *et al.*, 2013) 18 midwives were observed undertaking booking interviews with 34 women. Some midwives followed a structured format, tending to ask the questions directly; others appeared more sensitive and had a flexible approach, sometimes modifying the questions. The researchers considered that modification of the questions may help women interpret and understand the question, but it may also be due to the midwife feeling uncomfortable asking these sensitive questions and detract from the integrity of the assessment. So, let us now consider how different approaches may come across.

Activity 6.3   *Reflection*

How a midwife asks these sensitive questions is varied. Consider the following three options: 'Have you ever had mental health issues?' 'May I ask if you have had serious depression, schizophrenia, bipolar disorder or psychosis or other serious mental illness?' Or 'Have you been feeling flat, low or down lately?' Which form of the question do you think is most appropriate and why? Discuss this with one of your peers on the course. What other ways have you heard midwives ask these questions?

Suggested answers will be at the end of the chapter.

The manner in which these personal questions are asked may affect the responses women give. Historically mental illness has been stigmatised; this means that a label of difference is sometimes applied and the stigma of the illness and negative connotations associated with having a particular illness can overshadow the rest of the person's life, or in this case the pregnancy. Thus some women may not disclose previous or present mental illness, for fear of being labelled. Therefore all midwives have a responsibility both to ask the questions as sensitively as possible, and to articulate what specific illnesses they are looking to identify, otherwise the non-disclosure may be about misunderstanding the question as opposed to the women not wanting to discuss their history.

A systematic review (Lancaster *et al.*, 2010), which is a literature review which synthesises high quality research, identified risk factors associated with antenatal depression. (While we are trying not to separate antenatal and postnatal perinatal illness, you will see later in this chapter that the factors associated in this list also affect women after birth, which reinforces the view that the whole pregnancy and childbearing period should be assessed.) The following factors were seen as contributory: maternal anxiety, life stress, prior depression, lack of social support, domestic violence, unintended pregnancy and relationship factors (Lancaster *et al.*, 2010).

Activity 6.4   *Critical thinking*

Using the list: maternal anxiety, life stress, prior depression, lack of social support, domestic violence, unintended pregnancy and relationship factors, can you separate these into social and psychological factors? Discuss with a friend to see if your lists compare. Are there any factors missing from this list that you think are associated with perinatal depression or mental illness?

The next paragraph will offer the answer.

From this list you can see it takes some thought to categorise these into psychological and social factors. The psychological factors are previous or present anxiety or depression and/or stressful life events such as divorce, or death of a loved one. The social factors are related to support from the woman's partner and relatives and pregnancy intent. The association of domestic abuse to antepartum depression could be seen as both social, because it involves an intimate partner, and psychological, since it will impact upon the woman's mental wellbeing. While these factors should not be used in isolation to predict the development of a mental disorder, they may be used in conjunction with the above prediction and detection (Whooley) questions and may help you understand perinatal mental illness.

Missing from the Lancaster *et al.* (2010) list is the association between poverty, deprivation and perinatal mental illness. The link between poverty and poor general and mental health is well-known, but difficult to understand fully. The link may be bi-directional, which means it works both ways; people who are poor may have poor mental health, but having poor mental health may affect your income and you will become poor. As a midwife you must not be judgemental in your approach to women and their families, and while there are links between poverty and poor mental health, living in a deprived area alone is not a sign of mental illness and people with mental illness do not all live in poor circumstances. So again poverty should not be used in isolation, but an understanding of the impact of poverty and its association with poor mental health may help you identify women who may need extra social or psychological support. It is the psychological support this chapter is focusing on.

In the latest NICE (2014c) guidance screening for postnatal mental health problems is associated with higher risk for certain groups of women. These women are those who smoke; have high or low body mass, which may be associated with a mental health disorder; who self-harm or neglect themselves; consume alcohol or illicit drugs; live in poor relationships; experience domestic abuse; are socially isolated or have housing, immigration or economic status problems; basically all those groups of women who are covered by the chapters of this book.

Documentation and communication of assessment

If the woman has a history of previous *mild or moderate* mental illness an individualised care plan should be written in partnership with the woman and her family. For the first time the new NICE guidance (2014c) offers a further category of health assessment; for women who have a low mood but do not have a diagnosis of mild or moderate illness a referral to their GP for further support in the first instance is recommended. Any of these classifications would enable you the midwife to refer the woman to services to support her care; in the first instance this is usually her GP.

If the woman has a *severe* mental illness, she should be referred urgently to a specialist mental health service (NICE, 2014c). The woman's GP should be informed in all cases, whether treatment is required or not. If the midwife identifies a woman who needs further care, it is the midwife's role to ensure this referral and communication process occurs. The reasons for such prompt referrals and the responsibility for following this up has arisen from previous reports from the Centre for Maternal and Child Enquiries (CMACE) formerly called the Confidential Enquiry into Maternal and Child Health (CEMACH) which showed women died because serious mental illness concerns were not followed up promptly, and the care many of the women received was substandard. For every woman who dies, lessons should be learned so that care can be improved to prevent further maternal deaths. From 1 January 2013, the organisation Mothers and Babies: Reducing Risk through Audits and Confidential Enquiries across the UK (MBRRACE-UK) has been responsible for collecting national information about maternal deaths, as well as CMACE. The latest report (Knight *et al.*, 2014) shows the number of women who died from psychiatric disorders from 2010–2012 ($n = 16$), but the full report on these women's deaths is not due until later in 2015. The final section of this chapter will consider maternal suicide, but first the need to recognise common mental health disorders.

Common mental health disorders

Now you have considered some of the terms used in this chapter and the importance of early identification of risk for all women, we will continue with a brief overview of common mental health disorders. Common mental disorders are mental conditions that cause marked emotional distress and interfere with daily function, but do not usually affect insight or cognition (they do not alter the person's thought processes). These are considered to be depression and anxiety. The prevalence of depression and anxiety is as the name suggests common; approximately one woman in five and one man in eight have these disorders (McManus *et al.*, 2009).

Generalised anxiety disorders can exist in isolation, but more commonly occur with other anxiety and depressive disorders. Therefore there is some difficulty in diagnosing and treating disorders,

Disorder	Definition	Symptoms	Impact
Depression	Characterised by an absence of a positive mood (NICE, 2011).	Tearfulness, irritation with others, and withdrawal from social life, fatigue, loss of sexual desire, reduced sleep and lower appetite.	It may be harder for people with depression to concentrate and they may remember negative experiences more vividly than other people. The average age of the first depressive episode is mid-20s, although this can manifest in childhood or adolescence.
Anxiety is an umbrella term and includes other named disorders: generalised anxiety disorder (GAD), panic disorder, phobias, social anxiety disorder, obsessive-compulsive disorder (OCD) and post-traumatic stress disorder (PTSD) (NICE, 2011).			
Generalised anxiety disorders	Excessive worry on most days for at least six months (NICE, 2011).	Anxiety is difficult to control and the person is frequently restless, easily tired, and irritable and has disturbed sleep.	This may affect their normal routines. Generalised anxiety disorder is often a chronic condition, which means it is persistent and the rates of remission or recovery are low. The most common age of onset is mid-20s; however onset can occur at any age.
Panic disorders	Short-lived episodes of anxiety.	Can lead onto agoraphobia, fear of being in a place or situation where it is difficult to leave and may result in social isolation, if the person cannot find a cause of the panic disorder.	The frequency and intensity of the panic varies.
Obsessive-compulsive disorders	The presence of an obsession or compulsion, but often both.	An obsession is an unwelcome thought or image which manifests in the person's mind that can be distressing. A compulsion is a repeated behaviour that the person feels obligated to perform.	Compulsions can be excessive cleaning and checking, but many other presentations exist. For women the mean age of obsessive-compulsive disorders is early 20s; it may take individuals between 10–15 years to seek professional help.

(Continued)

(Continued)

Disorder	Definition	Symptoms	Impact
Post-traumatic stress disorder	Often develops after a traumatic life event; these can be accidents, natural disasters or personal disasters such as violence or abuse.	The specific symptoms of PTSD can vary widely between individuals, but they generally fall into the categories of re-experiencing a trauma, avoidance of events and reminders of the trauma and hyper arousal. Depression, anxiety and drug or alcohol misuse are often experienced too.	The memory of the trauma is often re-lived and the symptoms experienced at the time are re-experienced.
Social anxiety disorder or social phobia	Fear of social situations.	Extreme sweating, blushing, trembling, palpitations and nausea.	This fear impacts upon the person causing them distress. They can feel judged by others, extreme embarrassment or humiliation. This then leads to avoiding the social situation.
Specific phobias	Can be associated with animals, blood, storms, transport or other fears.	The phobia is an extreme fear that is out of proportion to the actual danger.	Phobia can interfere with everyday life as the person attempts to avoid exposure to their fear.

Table 6.3: Mild and moderate mental illnesses

and anxiety can often be under-detected. Depression affects social and physical functioning, so women with depression may not be able to look after themselves. Normal pregnancy changes, such as increase or loss of appetite, may also be a symptom of a mental health problem. Women may not eat or they may binge eat; they may not be able to sleep well, and this has an impact upon the developing fetus and baby once born.

The key message from this brief resume of the mild and moderate mental health disorders is that they are common in the general population and in pregnancy. You will also note that many of these illnesses manifest in the 20s; as the average age of a first pregnancy is late 20s, many women will either have a history of these mild or moderate illnesses or they manifest at the time of the pregnancy.

Severe mental illness

Severe mental illness is less common. The severe disorders are often termed psychoses. The difference between the mild and moderate or severe illness is the loss of rational thought in psychotic disorders. The main severe disorders are schizophrenia, mood disorders, such as bipolar disorder, and severe depression.

	Definition	Symptoms	Impact
Schizophrenia	A disorder of the mind that affects how you think, feel and behave.	Hallucinations: hearing, smelling, feeling or seeing something – but it isn't caused by anything (or anybody) around you. Delusions: believing something strongly, while others disagree. Thought disorders, being controlled, paranoid. Losing interest in life, appearance, concentration. Associated with depression (50%).	Onset 15–35 years, affects men and women equally, more common in cities and some ethnic groups. Affects 1 in 100 people, but if a parent or sibling are affected this rises to 1 in 10.
Bipolar disorder	Condition in which the mood can swing very high or low for weeks or months at a time.	Low mood with intense depression and despair. High or 'manic' mood with elation, over-activity or anger. A 'mixed state' with symptoms of depression and mania.	Affects 1 in 100 people, seems to run in families. Rate of relapse higher in postnatal period. May also present as a first occurrence in postnatal period.
Severe depression	Low mood for a prolonged period.	Hard to make decisions, loss of interest in life, sex, low self-confidence, and appetite, feels tired, restless, agitated.	One in five people will become depressed; four out of five will recover without treatment in 4–6 months. One in five will still be depressed 2 years later. If you have one episode of depression, there is a 50% chance of it reoccurring.

Table 6.4: Severe mental disorders

Ongoing midwifery care

While the beginning of this chapter considered the midwife's responsibility at the first contact with the woman, throughout her pregnancy, at each antenatal appointment, you, the midwife, should be assessing the woman's mood and risk factors. Both these, mood and risk factors, can change during the pregnancy. You will already know if you have been out in practice, that women can have relationship breakdowns while pregnant, suffer the loss of a loved family member or friend, and experience other traumatic or stressful life events, which can impact on their mental health.

While the first consultation with the woman at the booking interview is an important stage in identifying and detecting women at greater risk, each appointment is an opportunity to assess women's mental health. If left untreated, moderate depression can develop into severe depression and, in a few cases, lead to maternal suicide.

The effects of perinatal mental illness are widespread. If we consider a case study you may be able to think about these effects.

Case study: Anxiety in pregnancy

At 28 weeks' gestation, Eliza expressed increasing backache, heartburn and tiredness to Cathy, her midwife. Cathy explained all these symptoms were normal, but continued to ask about how these symptoms were affecting Eliza. She explained these physical symptoms left her questioning her ability to cope with the rest of her pregnancy, and then the baby that would follow. Her ability to care for herself was affected as she was too tired to cook and eat well; her partner thought she was making a fuss and this was causing tension in their relationship. So Eliza said she spoke to him less as a result.

If you were Eliza's midwife, what would you feel she needs and why?

The text after this scenario will help link Eliza's needs to midwifery care discussions.

Cathy is able to see from Eliza's conversation that several issues are present. The symptoms of tiredness, back pain and heartburn are affecting Eliza's physical health. Her current mental health seems to be affected by these physical symptoms. Her adjustment to motherhood is worrying her. She is experiencing a lack of social support, as her partner does not understand her need for psychological support. This is leading to less interaction between the two of them and may further affect her mental and physical health and that of her fetus if she is or becomes depressed.

Women identified as suffering from current mild or moderate illness should be referred to their GP in the first instance (RCOG, 2011). For women who develop mild or moderate depression or anxiety in pregnancy, self-help strategies should be considered. These include guided self-help, cognitive behavioural therapy or exercise and peer support groups. Hopefully you know of some within your local area. Research (Jones *et al.*, 2014) explored the impact of peer support on the woman's emotional journey with perinatal mental illness. They found there were four themes in the way women move towards wellbeing: (1) 'Isolation: the role of peer support'; (2) 'Seeking validation through peer support'; (3) 'The importance of social norms of motherhood'; and (4) 'Finding affirmation/a way forward; the impact of peer support'. Recommendations from this research suggest practitioners should identify women who are isolated and help them develop their peer support networks. This strategy, along with a referral to her GP, may work for Eliza.

If there were other more severe symptoms identified in the antenatal period such as suicidal thoughts, self-neglect, evidence of harm or significant interference with daily functioning then an urgent referral to specialist perinatal mental health services or general psychiatric services would be required (RCOG, 2011). Women who present to the midwife with new symptoms in late pregnancy should be considered at high risk of perinatal mental illness.

Intrapartum care

If the antenatal assessments were thorough, there should be an agreed plan in place for the intrapartum period. This is only really pertinent to a woman with severe present mental illness. It will consider whether the woman can continue to take their prescribed (psychotropic) medication, and the impact of these on her analgesic and anaesthetic options and her neonate.

If we reconsider Eliza here, her physical symptoms remained problematic for her during the pregnancy. She was referred to her GP who recommended she attend a perinatal support group. This involved an assessment at home, a volunteer offering befriending visits and attendance at support groups. Eliza did not attend the support groups, but the befriending service enabled her to share her anxieties about the imminent arrival of the baby and she was encouraged to talk to her partner about these. As a result of these improved intimate conversations and more support from her partner, Eliza's mood improved during the pregnancy. She therefore had no plan of care implemented for the intrapartum period.

The postnatal period

The NICE (2014c) *Antenatal and Postnatal Mental Health Guidelines* remind practitioners to re-assess past or present mental health at the first contact in the postnatal period. For other women who have not been previously affected by mental illness, social support should be offered by the midwife in the postnatal period. This includes asking the woman how she is feeling, coping and sleeping (NICE, 2014c). As you saw in the antenatal scenario, physical symptoms can affect mental health. Support can be offered individually; equally there are social support networks that a woman and her baby may access locally in a group format. These range from breastfeeding cafés to infant massage groups and are frequently offered in Children's Centres.

Women in the postnatal period may experience a mild, moderate or severe mood disorder. This chapter has already mentioned the pre-existing common and less common disorders; these may manifest as a first occurrence, or as a re-occurrence. There are also some other emotional responses to pregnancy and birth and these will be considered now.

The period after birth has been associated with the 'baby blues'. This is a normal physiological phenomenon experienced by as many as 80% of women postnatally in the first week after birth. It manifests as tearfulness which needs no treatment and is self-limiting; it resolves in a few days. It typically occurs on the 3–4th day after birth and resolves within 48 hours. The midwife's role includes asking women the Whooley questions; asking about their social support and reassuring women that these symptoms are normal for the majority of women. You will

	Incidence and manifestation	Signs and symptoms	Midwife's role
Birth trauma	Many women experience a birth that is not what they expected. This can manifest in transient disappointment but for some women it can lead to post-traumatic stress disorder (2–7% of births).	Intrusion of thoughts, memories or flashbacks to the distressing event. Avoidance of reminders, similar situations or events related to the distressing event. More likely to develop in a woman with a history of previous mental illness.	Identify women at risk, refer to GP. Cognitive behavioural therapies may help. Liaise with health visitor.
Mild or moderate depression	The prevalence of depression in the postnatal period ranges from 3% to 25% across studies. The first 3 months after birth is the period of highest risk of developing mild or moderate depression.	Depressive mood, anhedonia (inability to feel pleasure), anxiety, irritability, insomnia, lack of appetite, tiredness, tearfulness, low self-esteem, feelings of inadequacy or guilt, and thoughts of self-harm or suicide.	Ask Whooley questions, recognise signs and symptoms, refer to GP. Longer period of postnatal visiting by midwife may help support mother–baby relationship development. Liaise with health visitor. Offer postnatal support groups or peer support. With treatment symptoms usually reduce and recovery by 6 months is likely.
Severe depressive illness	Prevalence around 3% of women, onset gradual in first 2–12 weeks.	Emotional detachment and low mood, loss of appetite and then weight, poor concentration, fearfulness, agitation and restlessness, lethargy, broken sleep patterns, loss of pleasure; some mothers may be unable to care for their baby, others may be fiercely protective of theirs.	Refer to GP and psychiatric services. Continue to support mother and family. Share information with health visitor.
Puerperal or postpartum psychosis	It is a severe episode of mental illness which begins suddenly, usually in the 2–7 days after having a baby. It occurs in about two in every 1000 women (0.2%) who have a baby.	High mood (mania), depression, confusion, hallucinations and delusions, agitation, restlessness, suspiciousness and a sense of foreboding may occur. Symptoms vary and can change rapidly.	Postpartum psychosis is a psychiatric emergency. You should seek help as quickly as possible. Admission to a specialist perinatal mother and baby unit is considered the optimal care.

Table 6.5: Identifying postnatal mental illness

though be vigilant in the postnatal period and recognise those women whose symptoms do not resolve in 48 hours. These women will need a referral to either their GP or specialist perinatal psychiatric services. Table 6.5 will help you see who needs further care.

It has been debated whether puerperal psychosis and postnatal depression are separate psychiatric disorders, or whether pregnancy and birth are such stressful events for some women that severe psychotic or depressive events can manifest in vulnerable women following birth (Price, 2007). Whatever the cause women need prompt recognition and referral to appropriate services if they exhibit signs and symptoms of mild, moderate or severe mental illness. A midwife's role in the postnatal period is to support the infant–mother relationship and to detect deviations from the normal patterns. When a deviation is detected appropriate referrals must be made. At least half of women who give birth express low mood at some time during their pregnancy or postnatally (SIGN, 2012). Symptoms include feeling overwhelmed and tearful, but these may pass with rest and support. The midwife has to differentiate between normal symptoms and those which indicate more serious depressive illness.

Case study: After the birth

The day following the normal birth of their daughter, Grace, the family returned home. Eliza struggled with breastfeeding for the first four days. Her midwife, Cathy, attended each day to support Eliza. Every day she was tearful, but determined to feed. The midwifery support worker or breastfeeding supporter also visited Eliza. Eventually Grace managed to latch onto the breast and feed, albeit for short periods. On the 5th day when Grace was weighed she had lost 10% of her birth weight. The local guidelines suggested giving Grace supplementary formula milk to prevent further weight loss. Knowing Eliza's previous history, Cathy was worried that undermining her confidence and ability to breastfeed Grace might cause Eliza distress. She had a frank conversation with Eliza and her partner about the need for Grace to regain some of her birth weight and the importance of Eliza to rest for the next 24 hours to be able to supply and offer Grace feeds each time she demonstrated feeding cues and express milk from her breasts to supplement Grace's intake. Cathy explained the family could supplement Eliza with formula feeds, but it was their decision. Eliza was less tearful as she thought the breastfeeding was starting to get better and really wanted to be able to feed. The following day Eliza reported that the feeding had really improved over the last 24 hours, and when Grace was weighed she had begun to gain weight. Cathy kept visiting Eliza until day 12 when her care was handed over to the health visitor. There were no further concerns about Eliza's mental health.

Case study: Another midwife, another outcome

Imagine that instead of continuing her postnatal care with Cathy, another midwife who has not met Eliza before and does not know her history takes over the postnatal visits from day 5. This midwife says Grace needs supplementary formula feeds because of her weight loss. Eliza is tearful as she is disappointed, but understands the advice. The parents give Grace artificial milk; she sleeps for 3 hours and

continued . . .

continued . . .

> *when she wakes it is hard for her to latch to the breast as it is so full. So the parents decide she better have another bottle. The cycle continues, and by the morning Grace's weight is improved, but Eliza is feeling sad she has not been able to feed her. There is limited opportunity for Eliza to express this to her midwife, so she says nothing. When care of Grace is handed over to the health visitor on day 12, she is being fed exclusively with formula milk. There are concerns about Eliza's attachment to Grace.*

If left untreated, the maternal morbidity will continue for longer than with treatment and maternal mortality may occur. While maternal suicide is rare it is still one of the biggest causes of maternal death and may be preventable. The Centre for Maternal and Child Enquiries (CMACE) published a detailed 3-yearly report in 2011, stating the number of women who died directly, or indirectly, during or after their pregnancy. The number of women who died in that triennium, three years, from 2006–2008, related to perinatal mental health, was 41 with 29 women due to suicide. Sixteen of these women took their lives after giving birth, so there were 13 suicides during the pregnancy. 'Over half of the maternal suicides were White, married, employed women living in comfortable circumstances and aged 30 years or older' (CMACE, 2011). Therefore suicide is an example of where care needs to be taken that midwives do not associate the risk with socioeconomic deprivation. All the women who died had symptoms of psychiatric disorder, whether this was anxiety, depression or previous psychiatric disorders. Women with a significant previous diagnosis have a 50% risk of reoccurrence (CMACE, 2011). In 2015 a report by Mothers and Babies: Reducing Risk through Audits and Confidential Enquiries across the UK (MBRRACE-UK) will detail the 16 early (within 6 weeks of birth) and 95 late maternal deaths (from 6 weeks to 1 year following birth) due to psychiatric causes. To help you think about your own skills consider the next activity.

Activity 6.5   *Critical thinking*

Access the CMACE publication, in particular, Chapter 13 Midwifery. It can be found here: **http://onlinelibrary.wiley.com/doi/10.1111/j.1471-0528.2010.02847.x/abstract**

Reflect on what skills you need to improve to ensure you can learn from this substandard care.

As this is about your own skills, there is no suggested answer at the end of the chapter.

Now you have considered the CMACE recommendations, care of the neonate will be considered in relation to maternal mental illness.

Postnatal neonatal care

Infants of women who have taken psychotropic medication in pregnancy will be observed for signs of neonatal abstinence or adaption syndrome (or signs of withdrawal) in the early postnatal period. The neonate can demonstrate neurobehavioural signs that are symptomatic of exposure to drugs such as psychotropic medications in pregnancy. These include insomnia, poor feeding, vomiting, diarrhoea, irritability, restlessness, poor temperature control, tachypnoea and seizures. The observations can occur on the postnatal ward, so the mother and baby are not separated initially, but if signs of neonatal adaption syndrome occur, the baby will be transferred for care to a neonatal unit. The signs and symptoms usually occur within the first 3 days and may resolve spontaneously; breastfeeding may help reduce the symptoms as small amounts of the drug will be excreted in the breastmilk. Occasionally medication is given to the baby to alleviate symptoms, but all babies should be observed.

The effects of maternal mental illness on the neonate range from an inability of the mother to complete small day-to-day tasks to unintended neglect of their baby. Similarly lack of pleasure in the baby may be the cause or result of mental illness; an unsettled crying baby who is difficult to feed and comfort may exacerbate mild depressive illness or be the cause of mild illness. The long-term effects of maternal mental illness include attachment disorders and reduced cognitive ability as the child develops. Again, with prompt recognition and referral, treatment can be initiated to the mother and the effects on the mother, infant and the family can be minimised.

Case study: Supporting Eliza

If we return to Eliza and Grace, in the scenario where there are concerns about Eliza's attachment to Grace, we will recognise that something needs to be done to support Eliza. Improving the attachment between mothers and babies can be supported with perinatal mental health services, similar to the antenatal support Eliza had (Coe and Barlow, 2013). Eliza may agree to have the befriending home visits again. She may this time agree to other support groups, or attend a local infant massage group to encourage a more positive interaction between her and Grace. Before Eliza can agree to any of these activities, the midwife or health visitor has to have the conversation with Eliza regarding their worries about her deteriorating mental health. They also have to refer their concerns to the GP. They can then offer services in the local area to support Eliza, according to her wishes. Left without support, Eliza's health may deteriorate and this will have consequences for Grace and Eliza's partner. Many women who agree to become a volunteer befriender have experienced low mood themselves and have a desire to 'give back' to their community. Their support may be enough to help Eliza find her internal resources to improve her interactions with Grace and her partner. If this does not happen the GP could consider medication for Eliza, but self-help strategies and regular support are often sufficient, if implemented early to improve women's and their babies' lives.

While there is a correlation between social and economic deprivation and the onset of perinatal mental illness, *any* woman can be affected by mental illness. The 2011 CMACE report showed there was, for the first time, a slight reduction in the number of women who died who also lived in deprivation, demonstrating a reduction in the gap between social groups; historically, those living in the most deprived areas had the highest rates of maternal morbidity. This is known as an inequality gap. Your role as a midwife is to predict and detect which women are at increased risk of mental illness and refer appropriately, so they are offered the most effective treatment and the long-term effects to themselves and their family are reduced.

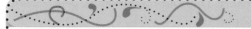

Chapter summary

This chapter introduced the care of the woman and her family regarding the identification and referral process in relation to perinatal mental illness. The importance of early detection, through the Whooley questions at the booking interview, in conjunction with awareness of a woman's altered mood in pregnancy is imperative. The two new NICE (2014c) questions to detect often overlooked anxiety were introduced. The categorisation of perinatal mental illness as mild, moderate and severe helps the midwife decide who she needs to inform regarding the woman's ongoing care. The availability of local voluntary agencies as well as professional services to support and treat women with perinatal mental health problems has been considered. For this chapter to make more sense, you need to find out the local services and referral pathways in your area to fully support women. Being attentive to their needs is the first step, but practical ongoing support is needed to improve their lives and that of their families.

Activities: brief outline answer

Activity 6.3 Reflection [page 104]

The NICE (antenatal guidance) says midwives should use the Whooley questions, the third question in the activity AND ask about the woman's past or present mental health; therefore a form of question 1 and/or 2 should be used with question 3. Question 1 may seem more abrupt, but question 2 may be too specific for some midwives to ask.

Further reading

All of the below are recommended documents that will support your knowledge development of common mental health disorders and care decisions.

NICE (2004a) *Anxiety: Management of Anxiety (Panic Disorder, With or Without Agoraphobia, and Generalised Anxiety Disorder) in Adults in Primary, Secondary and Community Care.* NICE Clinical Guideline 22. Available at: **www.nice.org.uk/CG22**

NICE (2004b) *Self-Harm: the Short-Term Physical and Psychological Management and Secondary Prevention of Self-Harm in Primary and Secondary Care.* NICE Clinical Guideline 16. Available at: **www.nice.org. uk/CG16**

NICE (2005a) *Obsessive-Compulsive Disorder: Core Interventions in the Treatment of Obsessive-Compulsive Disorder and Body Dysmorphic Disorder.* NICE Clinical Guideline 31. Available at: **www.nice.org.uk/ CG31**

NICE (2005b) *Post-traumatic Stress Disorder (PTSD): the Management of PTSD in Adults and Children in Primary and Secondary Care.* NICE Clinical Guideline 26. Available at: **www.nice.org.uk/CG26**

NICE (2006) *Bipolar Disorder: the Management of Bipolar Disorder in Adults, Children and Adolescents, in Primary and Secondary Care.* NICE Clinical Guideline 38. Available at: **www.nice.org.uk/CG38**

NICE (2007) *Antenatal and Postnatal Mental Health: Clinical Management and Service Guidance.* NICE Clinical Guideline 45. Available at: **www.nice.org.uk/CG45**

NICE (2009) *Depression: the Treatment and Management of Depression in Adults.* NICE Clinical Guideline 90. Available at: **www.nice.org.uk/CG90**

NICE (2011) *Generalised Anxiety Disorder and Panic Disorder (With or Without Agoraphobia) in Adults: Management in Primary, Secondary and Community Care.* NICE Clinical Guideline 113. Available at: **www.nice.org.uk/CG113**

NICE (2013) *Social Anxiety Disorder: Recognition, Assessment and Treatment.* NICE Clinical Guideline 159. Available at: **www.nice.org.uk/CG159**

Useful websites

Action on Postpartum Psychosis

www.app-network.org

A patient organisation aimed at building up a pool of women who have experienced postpartum psychosis and are interested in helping with research. Aims to provide up-to-date research information to women who have experienced postpartum psychosis and their families.

Association for Post-Natal Illness (APNI)

www.apni.org

APNI is a charity which provides information and support to anyone affected by postnatal depression. Information leaflets can be downloaded from the website.

Child and Maternal Health Intelligence Network

www.chimat.org.uk

A dedicated team providing health intelligence, knowledge management and support to practitioners in the field.

Since 1 April 2013, the former Child and Maternal Health Observatory (ChiMat) has been part of Public Health England (PHE), an executive agency of the Department of Health. PHE has been established to protect and improve the nation's health and wellbeing and to reduce inequalities. This website continues to be updated.

Has a particularly good section on mental health and psychological wellbeing.

Chapter 7
Domestic abuse

Helen Muscat

Practise in a way which respects, promotes and supports individuals' rights, interests, preferences, beliefs and cultures. This will include:

- offering culturally sensitive family planning advice;
- ensuring that women's labour is consistent with their religious and cultural beliefs and preferences;
- the different roles and relationships in families, and reflecting different religious and cultural beliefs, preferences and experiences.

Practise in accordance with relevant legislation. This will include:

- practising within the contemporary legal framework of midwifery;
- demonstrating knowledge of legislation relating to human rights, equal opportunities, equality and diversity, and access to client records;
- demonstrating knowledge of legislation relating to health and social policy relevant to midwifery practice;
- demonstrating knowledge of contemporary ethical issues and their impact on midwifery practice.
- Managing the complexities arising from ethical and legal dilemmas.

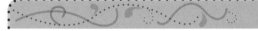

NMC Essential Skills Clusters

This chapter will address the following ESCs:

Cluster: Communication:

5. Treat women with dignity and respect them as individuals.
6. Work in partnership with women in a manner that is diversity sensitive and is free from discrimination, harassment and exploitation.
7. Provide care that is delivered in a warm, sensitive and compassionate way.
8. Be confident in their own role within a multidisciplinary/multi-agency team.

Chapter aims

By the end of this chapter you will have:

- gained a clear understanding of the midwife's role in addressing domestic abuse;
- challenged your professional and personal thoughts and feelings about addressing this issue;
- developed your understanding of women's perspectives;
- considered the skills and strategies which lead to behaviour change in women experiencing domestic abuse.

Introduction

Domestic abuse has been widely acknowledged as an area of public health concern. The Home Office (2013) has updated its definition to incorporate other aspects of abuse, stating:

Any incident or pattern of incidents of controlling, coercive or threatening behaviour, violence or abuse between those aged 16 or over who are or have been intimate partners or family members regardless of gender or sexuality. This can encompass but is not limited to the following types of abuse:

- *psychological;*
- *physical;*
- *sexual;*
- *financial;*
- *emotional.*

Controlling behaviour is: a range of acts designed to make a person subordinate and/or dependent by isolating them from sources of support, exploiting their resources and capacities for personal gain, depriving them of the means needed for independence, resistance and escape and regulating their everyday behaviour.

Coercive behaviour is: an act or a pattern of acts of assault, threats, humiliation and intimidation or other abuse that is used to harm, punish, or frighten their victim.*

*This definition includes so called 'honour' based violence, female genital mutilation (FGM) and forced marriage, and is clear that victims are not confined to one gender or ethnic group.

Source: Home Office (2013)

The Home Office also stresses that, while this is not a legislative change, the rationale for the change in the definition is to send a clear message to the perpetrators that any kind of abuse is not acceptable.

Women's Aid outlines an analysis of ten separate domestic violence prevalence studies that found consistent findings: one in four women experience domestic violence over their lifetimes and between 6–10% of women suffer domestic violence in a given year (Council of Europe, 2002). The repercussions of domestic abuse can have a lifelong impact not only on the women but on their offspring too, for the midwife safeguarding the child's wellbeing is paramount. This is particularly so when considering that in the UK during 2012–2013, 76 women were killed by an intimate partner or ex-partner (ONS, 2014).

The British Crime Survey found that there were an estimated 12.9 million incidents of domestic violence acts (that constituted non-sexual threats or force) against women and 2.5 million against men in England and Wales in the year preceding interview (Walby and Allen, 2004).

Although domestic abuse occurs across all age ranges, Smith *et al.* (2011) recorded those women aged 16–24 were at great risk of abuse. Frequently, men who will become violent do not reveal this side of their personality until they have been in a relationship for a year or until the first pregnancy.

Walby and Allen (2004) reporting on the British Crime Survey found that the first incident of domestic abuse, for 51% of the women, occurred one year or more into the relationship; for 30% of the women it occurred between three months and one year; and for 13% it was between one and three months. It occurred in less than one month for only 6% of women. Among a group of pregnant women attending primary care in East London, 15% reported violence during their pregnancy; just under 40% reported that violence started while they were pregnant, whereas 30% who reported violence during pregnancy also reported they had at some time suffered a miscarriage as a result (Coid, 2006).

In a study of 200 women's experiences of domestic violence it was found that 60% of the women had left because they feared that they or their children would be killed by the perpetrator (Humphreys and Thiara, 2002). Therefore it is reasonable to surmise that midwives will meet some of these women in maternity services.

Activity 7.1   *Critical thinking and group work*

Consider the types of abuse outlined in the Home Office definition above and discuss with two or three of your peers the types of events/incidents which may occur within these headings. Consider the words women may use to describe these to you.

As this is activity is concerned with your own experience and that of your peers, there is no outline answer at the end of the chapter.

What is the midwife's role in addressing domestic abuse?

The NMC makes clear that promoting health is an interprofessional concern (NMC, 2015), therefore your primary role as a healthcare professional may be identifying sufferers of abuse rather than resolving issues (Midwifery 2020, 2012). However, midwives may find incorporating appropriate questions into their interactions with women challenging, particularly if referral to another professional seems to be called for.

Empowerment

Let's explore your understanding of empowerment. The term has become something of a buzz word used within practice. Sometimes it even sounds like a task, for example: 'the midwife's role is to empower women.' Empowerment is a concept that should be embraced by midwives certainly because it reflects the ideology of midwifery practice: that midwives work in partnership with women, helping them to exercise choice and control over their birthing experience (Hunt and Symonds, 1995). This is greatly preferable to the paternalistic approach in which healthcare professionals take a 'top down approach' to public health (Laverack, 2005).

The word 'empowerment' can be literally defined as follows:

1. To invest with power, especially legal power or official authority.

2. To equip or supply with an ability; enable.

(Free Dictionary, 2013)

A key word in this definition is 'enable'. A midwife who enables successfully is a good facilitator. In order to achieve this, midwives must equip themselves with the tools to understand, address and facilitate. However, the woman must also be a willing participant, wanting to work in partnership with the midwife. The midwife must, in the case of domestic abuse, appreciate the nature of the perpetrator's strategies to dis-empower and take control over the woman's being; this may prevent her from joining in the process of empowerment as she feels powerless to do so. If this is the case, it raises the question: how can you actually contribute to the empowerment of this woman? It may mean that the summation of your care is just to listen, with no other action. This can be challenging on several levels. On a human level, there is a desire to remedy and rescue. Midwives are often natural 'doers' so it can be hard to listen to a woman's story of abuse and feel you are just walking away. It could be that the woman's experience has elements which mirror your own life experiences. This can raise a mixture of emotions that can encroach into your working day and be difficult to deal with.

Case study: Jenny

Jenny and Peter attend a booking interview during week 15 of her pregnancy. Sandra the midwife notes that Jenny is booking later than the recommended 10 weeks. However, Jenny and Peter explain that they weren't expecting this pregnancy to happen so soon into their relationship. Peter tells Sandra that their relationship started 10 months ago and he moved into her house after 6 weeks of knowing Jenny. He describes her as the love of his life and that he is thrilled about the baby. The couple sit close together and gaze into one another's eyes throughout the booking appointment; this make Sandra feels a little uncomfortable. Jenny seems a little shy and often refers to Peter for answers to routine questions. As the meeting progresses Sandra becomes concerned that Jenny isn't able to express herself and is in fact anxious about providing answers to the questions. Towards the end of the appointment Sandra gathers the hand-held notes, blood and scan forms and leaflets together. She reiterates the function and content of each, including the women's aid leaflet about domestic abuse.

It is vital that during your career you consider how empowered you feel, and what dis-empowers you. If you want to be effective in promoting health through empowerment sometimes it is advantageous to reflect on the things that make you feel dis-empowered and what are the strategies that can deal with this. This is self-empowerment; it can be as simple as writing the problem out and creating an action plan, or involve more complex strategies that could include counselling therapies and self-help.

Create two lists, one of the times you have felt dis-empowered and the other the most empowered times; they can relate to both professional and personal life.

As this is activity is concerned with your own ideas and experience, there is no outline answer at the end of the chapter.

The woman's perspective

Perhaps you should consider your intentions at this point; it is clear that all women should be asked about domestic abuse and whether it has occurred at some point in their life. In Jenny's case, you may feel that there is a stronger rationale for asking such questions because her behaviour triggers questions in your mind. It is important to consider that you may be the first person to whom a woman in your care has told her story of abuse to; perhaps you will be the last person she tells before she changes her situation, or is it that she wants to share her story of making the change but feels afraid that she may return to that environment because she feels vulnerable during the pregnancy?

If your intention is to facilitate some level of empowerment, it is important to understand the woman's health beliefs and their ability to change their circumstances. One way to achieve this is to utilise the Stages of Change Model (Prochaska and Velicer, 1997) as a point of reference.

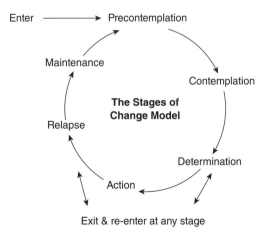

Figure 7.1: The Stages of Change Model. (http://sphweb.bumc.bu.edu/otlt/MPH-Modules/SB/SB721-Models/SB721-Models6.html)

The core foundation of this model is the process of change, that is the way we move through change, both explicitly and surreptitiously. The balance of decision-making is about how we come to a decision, weighing up the odds, how we cope with 'situations' and how we may live with an uncontrollable draw to a unhealthy habit or situation. The model itself begins with a pre-contemplation stage; during this stage the woman will not be considering a change to her life and may have negotiated a state that allows her to believe the circumstances are acceptable.

Laverack (2005) outlines three areas that the midwife could focus on to engage the woman in the process of empowering health choices:

1. Developing skills as an effective communicator.
2. Increasing the critical awareness of the woman.
3. Fostering an empowering professional–client relationship.

The model moves forward to a contemplation stage. This is the time when the midwife will have a huge impact on the thoughts and feelings that the woman is sharing. During this stage she may be considering how her lifestyle is impacting on the health and wellbeing of others. At this stage she will take on board some of the suggestions for reading literature and the thoughts of others, bearing in mind that the perpetrator will more than likely have isolated her socially and she may not have any one else to discuss these issues with. At this time the midwife can provide information, perhaps using written and verbal backup and resources outside of health such as women's aid and local helplines. It is vital that the woman does not feel pressurised to take information or call helplines at this time. It must be about information providing, choice and support.

The determination stage of the change cycle is the time to consider preparation: as a midwife you can gain a clear understanding of local resources and networks available to the woman. Perhaps it will be appropriate to discuss whether she is preparing to make a change to her circumstances, and what strategies might be helpful. Possibly this is the time to consider that the changes the woman may be considering to make to her lifestyle may not be as positive as you might hope. An example of this would be that from your perspective leaving the marital home would be the optimal change for the woman; however, it may be more realistic for the woman to develop strategies that will provide protection for her and the children/newborn.

Moving forward into the action stage, this is where the woman has the greatest risk of relapse. It is during this time she is also at the most danger. It is estimated that two women a week are killed by an intimate partner or ex-partner and it normally occurs during times of estrangement (Hunt and Martin, 2001). It is during such times that women are often intimidated and stalked by the abuser. Humphreys and Thiara (2002) identified that during this period 76% of separated women reported suffering post-separation violence.

Of these women:

*   76% were subjected to continued verbal and emotional abuse;
*   41% were subjected to serious threats towards themselves or their children;
*   23% were subjected to physical violence;
*   6% were subjected to sexual violence;
*   36% stated that this violence was ongoing.

This sort of pressure, particularly during pregnancy, can be exhausting and lead to feelings of dis-empowerment and the feeling that returning to the environment of abuse is preferable to being alone.

This relapse represents the final stage of the cycle, and it is estimated that women will leave an average of ten times before finalising the move.

So what is the midwife's role during these final two stages – action and relapse? The woman may only want a listening ear; she may require discussion and the development of a plan during the birth of her baby and thereafter. The plan you devise should be SMART in its approach. SMART goal are often associated with business or the employee targets for work. However, Haughney (2012) suggests this acronym can be altered to allow it to be utilised in other areas:

S – Significant

M – Motivational

A – Agreed upon and achievable

R – Realistic

T – Time-based

This provides a broader definition that will help you keep focused when creating your plan.

Asking the question

There is much debate about when the midwife should ask questions about domestic violence. The NICE guidance on antenatal care (NICE, 2008) suggests that the advice of the key professional and governmental bodies recommend 'routine enquiry' about domestic violence for all women. However it does not suggest when this should be, although NHS Trusts often encourage it to be at the booking interview. It is debatable whether this is truly the most appropriate time to ask this question; do women feel able to tell a stranger this information at this early stage of the woman–midwife relationship? Some may wish to keep the situation private, whether it is because they are estranged from their partner or that they wish to maintain a certain level of appearances. In a quantitative study on domestic abuse of pregnant women, Keeling and Birch (2004) asked the question: 'Do you think it would be a good idea to give women the opportunity to discreetly identify to staff that they are experiencing domestic abuse?' None of the participants replied 'No' to this question, 83.5% replied 'Yes' and the rest made no comment. However they did not identify when would be the optimal time for this conversation to take place. Ultimately, you need to have a sense of seizing the moment, seeing an opening that will foster a meaningful conversation, rather than undertaking a tick box exercise.

Now you have explored the woman's perspective, this is a moment to stop and reflect on how you feel about such questioning.

Activity 7.3 — *Reflection*

Review the list below; identify and tick which of the professional and personal issues may relate to you.

Professional issue

How do I ask the question?

What if I offend the woman?

What if she doesn't want to see me after asking?

What if she says yes? What do I do next?

Who am I to say what decision to make?

Personal issues

What if the woman shouts at me?

What if I can't face asking?

What if it is the same as my own experiences?

What if she cries?

Why don't they just leave?

I don't understand why women live like this.

As this is a reflective exercise that is based on your personal and professional experiences, you should be able to answer the questions as you move through this chapter.

To be effective you must take a holistic approach when communicating. It is important to remember that the woman is making a judgement about how much information to give to you and how honest and open she feels she can be. Her decision is based on a complex dance of verbal and nonverbal exchange which as the healthcare professional you have some control over.

The first aspect to consider is the environment, and as acknowledged in all current literature, this environment should be private and relaxed. In real terms this is not always reflected in the experience of midwifery practice today. Therefore, you should consider how to make the most of the surroundings you have. Try to undertake the booking in the woman's home or if you have booking clinics, consider how the desk and chairs are positioned: are you too close, will the position of the chairs invade her personal space? Could you alter the environment to be a bit more relaxed?

You should think about your facial expression and how you hold your body; arms folded is a closed body language that is often seen as defensive; fiddling with a pen or stethoscope will distract the woman from her thoughts. She may not make direct eye contact with you while replying to your questions. This is often because people are thinking and recalling information. As the listener you should continue to look at the woman, however, because if you are looking elsewhere when she does look at you, that will imply lack of commitment to the conversation (Scriven, 2010).

The next consideration is, how will you illicit the information needed to make a decision? Moss (2012) suggests that to encourage people to 'open up' open questions should be used. So what is an open question? When thinking about domestic abuse and questioning women, an example may be: What does your partner/husband think about this pregnancy?

It's important to remember that not everyone can open up, even if you have excellent communication skills. It can be that this issue evokes feeling of embarrassment, shame, sadness or fear. This is why the use of closed questions is equally important. It is often the closed question that midwives feel might provide a response they find difficult to deal with; an affirmative answer gives you time to think of a reply, but is it the answers of 'Why are you asking me?', 'Why should I tell you?', or even 'Mind your own business' that worry you? It is interesting to know that the evidence does not support midwives' fears. Women do want to share with their care provider; they do want to be believed and listened to (Keeling and Birch, 2004).

Activity 7.4   *Group working*

Get together with two or three other students and consider the definition of active listening; each jot down three words that describe this. Compare and discuss.

As this is activity is concerned with your own ideas and experience, there is no outline answer at the end of the chapter.

Active listening is not just about nodding at the right point. Trevithick (2010) outlined 20 basic skills involved in active listening and these incorporate the demonstration of your empathy, intuition and self-awareness. It suggests that not only should you be aware of your body language but demonstrate an understanding of the value of silence in the conversation and the emotion attached to the words. Moss (2012) describes this as listening to the music behind the words, stating that it is often the music that conveys the real meaning of the song.

An affirmative answer can be shocking; women's stories can be emotive, horrific and utterly heart-rending. Midwives are not immune to the feelings these stories evoke, which we will explore further in the chapter.

Remember that you must not agree to keep what you hear confidential from everyone; you are acting as a healthcare professional not as a friend, and that the wellbeing of the baby and other children remains paramount. This does not mean that you are not friendly, but be clear about your professional boundaries. However, it is crucial that you should acknowledge this disclosure in a way that the woman feels believed and validated. It may be appropriate to simply say that you appreciate how difficult it was to tell you this (Moss, 2012).

Let's explore the concept that is being suggested that you cannot keep a discussion confidential; the NMC Code (NMC, 2015) and Standards (NMC, 2012) charge nurses and midwives with the responsibility to respect a client's right to confidentiality and ensure they are fully informed. Should you need to share information, however, the codicil is if you believe the client or others may be at risk of harm, to have a responsibility to appropriately share such information. This really means sharing with an appropriate authority through the correct channels such as a Supervisor of Midwives or a manager.

'I just have a feeling'

Activity 7.5   *Research and evidence-based practice*

Consider the 'triggers' seen in the earlier case study and note what you may see in the following three aspects of the woman's care. Then develop this table to incorporate the wider 'triggers' that may be seen in general terms.

Obstetric wellbeing	Social wellbeing	Health behaviour

In order to complete this exercise, you should consider the signs and symptoms of domestic abuse and consider how these may present themselves in practice.

This article provides a clear overview:

Bacchus, L., Bewley, S. and Mezey, G. (2001) Domestic violence in pregnancy. *Fetal and Maternal Medicine Review*, 12: 249–271.

An outline answer to this activity is given at the end of this chapter.

Hunt and Martin (2001) suggest that an astute professional will link the physical signs to patterns of behaviours observed. The physical signs may be similar to those identified in Activity 7.2. You could relate this to the intuition of the midwife, knowing the behaviour of women; perhaps a better analogy is that of piecing a puzzle together. It is important that you do not jump to conclusions, that you build a picture of the woman's behaviour to gain a holistic overview of her situation. Consider her physical wellbeing, and her reactions such as anxiety, appearing frightened, interaction with healthcare provision and the explanation that goes with this. Sometimes this process does not occur at a conscious level; it is happening while you chat with her, or when you notice that she has not attended clinic again. It is at this point you have the 'choice' whether to suppress that 'feeling' or to consciously evaluate the situation and decide to take action. Women-centred midwifery campaigner Tricia Anderson coined the phrase 'drinking tea intelligently'. She applied the concept of looking like you're not doing much, but in your mind you are weighing up the pro and cons and making decisions. Although she applied this to normal birth, it can be applied to this interaction with a woman who is potentially in an abusive relationship. The woman will benefit from a midwife who not only focuses on her needs, looks calm, caring and empathetic, but professionally utilises that intuition to ignite a decision-making process that will benefit her care pathway.

Activity 7.6   *Reflection*

Revisit the list you previously identified in Activity 7.2. Re-evaluate, identify those you now feel reassured about and why this might be. For those that remain on your list, identify the barrier to moving forward with these and consider the strategies you may need to adopt to do so.

As this activity is concerned with your own ideas, thought and feelings, there is no outline answer at the end of the chapter.

Whatever the triggers are, and whenever or wherever you have the conversation with a woman about the possibility of abuse occurring in her life, as a midwife you will be making a judgement as to where she is in her own choices/option/decision-making processes. So let's go back to the Stages of Change cycle.

Activity 7.7   *Critical thinking*

www.youtube.com/watch?v=WvRGwmU4Qtg

Watch this clip and make notes: consider how this young woman moved through the Stages of Change Model and then consider why she told her story in written form rather than in person. Finally, consider why it is useful for you to know this?

As this activity is concerned with your own ideas, there is no outline answer at the end of the chapter.

Getting the answer to your questions

Allow the woman to complete her story – it is vital you acknowledge this and that you empathise with her experiences. This is a good time to take a deep breath and pause for a moment, as the most detrimental comment may be to ask, 'Why don't you leave?' Hunt and Martin (2001) also advise that the issue should not be reframed as an obstetric problem or mental health issue – it is a relationship issue.

Your response should relate to the woman's mindset, for example, if she is in the contemplation stage, you will give her different information than if she is in the action stage.

Activity 7.8   *Critical thinking*

Read the continuing scenario which explores Jenny's journey through pregnancy. Identify where you believe her to be in the Stages of Change Model and write down what your own reaction and actions might be. Consider the resources and advice you may be able to offer her.

continued . . .

continued . . .

> *Jenny is now in the 26th week of her pregnancy. During an antenatal visit Sandra notices she has a grip like bruise on the top of her arm. Sandra asks her directly about the bruises. Jenny begins to cry and says that Peter had done this. She explains that she had not been in on his return from work which had made him angry. He grabbed her by the arm as she tried to pass by him. Sandra states this is not okay for this to happen. Jenny stops crying, says she's just emotional and that it really wasn't that bad. Peter had apologised and was very sorry.*
>
> *Pre-contemplation*
>
> *Contemplation*
>
> *Determination*
>
> *Action*
>
> *Maintenance/relapse*
>
> *An outline answer to this activity is given at the end of this chapter.*

What next?

In this section, the care pathway for the woman has been divided into two categories: required and woman-led.

Once a disclosure has been acknowledged by you and you have paused to consider the way forward, your first thought should be about any immediate danger the woman is in. Of course not every type of abuse has physical elements and emotional abuse is very hard to respond to.

The safety plan can be simple suggestions and she may have already implemented them, but by verbalising a plan it allows you to reiterate their importance. Additionally, the conversation can be included in the woman's documentation. This should not be in the hand-held notes, in case the perpetrator reads this which may place her in a vulnerable situation. It should be in her hospital notes on a separate piece of paper, dated and signed.

Women's Aid (2013) provide suggestions for a safety plan that could include:

- Plan in advance how you might respond in different situations, including crisis situations.
- Think about the different options that may be available to you.
- Keep with you any important and emergency telephone numbers (for example, your local Women's Aid refuge organisation or other domestic violence service; the police domestic violence unit; your GP; your social worker, if you have one; your children's school; your solicitor).
- Teach your children to call 999 in an emergency and what they would need to say (for example, their full name, address and telephone number).
- Are there neighbours you could trust, and where you could go in an emergency? If so, tell them what is going on, and ask them to call the police if they hear sounds of a violent attack.

- Rehearse an escape plan, so in an emergency you and the children can get away safely.

- Pack an emergency bag for yourself and your children, and hide it somewhere safe (for example, at a neighbour's or friend's house). Try to avoid mutual friends or family.

- Try to keep a small amount of money on you at all times – including change for the phone and for bus fares.

- Know where the nearest phone is, and if you have a mobile phone, try to keep it with you.

- If you suspect that your partner is about to attack you, try to go to a lower risk area of the house – for example where there is a way out and access to a telephone. Avoid the kitchen or garage where there are likely to be knives or other weapons; and avoid rooms where you might be trapped, such as the bathroom, or where you might be shut into a cupboard or other small space.

- Be prepared to leave the house in an emergency.

Activity 7.9 — Decision-making

Look again at the suggestions from Women's Aid, above. Consider whether you could use these in practice. Could you adapt the list? Would it be useful to have as an aide memoire?

As this activity is concerned with your own ideas, there is no outline answer at the end of the chapter.

If discussing such a plan is not the most appropriate way forward at that moment, it may be a good time to ask the woman what she would like from you as her healthcare professional. This type of question has two benefits: it allows you to gain a clear idea of her expectations of you and then allows you to clearly clarify parameters and boundaries of your relationship. It is vital that you have this conversation; it helps to avoid any misunderstanding. At this point you should be clear what your role is and how far your sphere of practice extends. As this can be a very emotive time it is best to avoid words such as 'I promise' and beginning statements with 'I'm sure'. McBride (2002) discusses the client assessment of a substance user and highlights the need for the client to understand that at the very least the case will be discussed with a manager/supervisor and that you have a responsibility to work within the parameters of the Children's Act. This advice can be applied to the type of conversation you may have with abused women.

Activity 7.10 — Developing communication skills

Take a moment to reflect on your role here. Consider Jenny and how your relationship with her may have developed over the weeks. Plan how you would structure a conversation that includes a safety plan. It may be helpful to role play this with a fellow student.

Some suggested responses to this activity are given at the end of the chapter.

You may be asking yourself at this point of the conversation, 'Do I need social services input here?' There is no definite answer and each case must be judged on its own merits. You will have the opportunity to raise a cause for concern with social services; you are able to have a conversation with the agency and seek advice and direction. If you have any doubt, have the conversation! Remember that it is not just about the unborn baby, nor is it related to the type of abuse; consideration needs to be given to previous partners, other children and places of residence. As a midwife you have several directions you can move towards for support. You may have a team leader, matron or experienced buddy to ask initially for support. Consider the Named Midwife for child protection and locally the midwives she links with. Your Supervisor of Midwives (SOM) may be able to offer you time to discuss areas of conflict between personal and professional self. Additionally, the SOM may have a lateral view of the processes linked to domestic abuse and child protection, incorporating areas such as documentation.

Documenting abuse

At the beginning of this section it was stated that there would be two care pathways for women addressed here; the rationale for doing this is to add perspective to the issues of domestic abuse. For many women it is true they are physically abused and the interventions required may very well be affirmative and proactive. However, for an undisclosed number of women the abuse is insidious, difficult to pinpoint or address, yet it has an impact on their emotional and physical wellbeing. Their level of dis-empowerment and vulnerability is as great. Therefore, considering this, the question of 'What can I do for you?' is a vital component to the conversation. The answer is not easy, as 'just' listening can be frustrating for midwives; fixing situations in a proactive way is much more rewarding. You will still need to consider the issues of child protection, but may come to the conclusion there is no input required. You will still need to document the conversation in the main hospital notes as always, but any further action may be totally woman-led.

Your role as a healthcare professional

Documentation is intrinsic to the role of the midwife; however when documenting a disclosure of domestic abuse, you could consider including the following in the hospital notes as previously discussed, not hand-held notes:

- date of incident/s;
- time of incident/s;
- location of incident;
- name of abuser;
- what the woman states the abuser did to them, in their own words;
- how they felt as a result of the incident;
- list of witnesses, pictures, body map.

As a midwife, you have a responsibility to understand how your practice area communicates information between healthcare professionals; it may be that you have a sticker or tick box on the hand-held notes that identifies that there has been an affirmative answer to questions related to domestic abuse. If you are unsure, discuss it with your mentor, manager or a Supervisor of Midwives.

While it is acknowledged that as a midwife you cannot know everything about all subjects, having some idea about the key elements of domestic abuse will help advise and support women. For some midwives, they may feel this can become an area of expertise, therefore developing a scope of knowledge and understanding will help other midwives too.

Research summary: Domestic abuse

MARAC encompasses multi-agency risk assessment conferences which are multi-agency meetings of statutory and voluntary agency representatives such as police, social care, housing, education, health, probation services and victim support. They share information about high-risk victims of domestic abuse, developing action plans to increase victim safety. In 2011, approximately 250 MARACs were identified in England and Wales (Steel *et al.*, 2011).

Co-ordinated Action against Domestic Abuse (CAADA) is a charitable organisation that supports the MARAC process in England and Wales. They provide co-ordination for domestic abuse resources, have a MARAC database and provide telephone support along with an e-newsletter. All localities in the UK have a MARAC development officer allocated to provide such services. Seek out your local MARAC group and review the work they have undertaken locally.

The bills and legislations related to the abuse of women are available on the government website (**www.gov.uk**) with amendments and full copies of the Act with explanatory notes available.

Commonly referred Acts include: the Domestic Violence, Crime and Victims Act 2004; The Female Genital Mutilation (FGM) Act which:

- makes it illegal to practise FGM in the UK;
- makes it illegal to take girls who are British nationals or permanent residents of the UK abroad for FGM whether or not it is lawful in that country;
- makes it illegal to aid, abet, counsel or procure the carrying out of FGM abroad;
- has a penalty of up to 14 years in prison and, or, a fine.

The recently updated Protection from Harassment Act 1997 was updated by provisions made in the Protection of Freedoms Act 2012, creating two new offences for stalking, namely:

- stalking;
- stalking involving fear of violence or serious alarm and distress.

These amendments also provide the police with powers to enter and search premises with a warrant.

Activity 7.11   *Research and evidence-based practice*

Take a look at these websites and reflect upon the usefulness to women who find themselves in an abusive relationship while they are pregnant.

www.womensaid.org.uk

www.ncdv.org.uk

www.refuge.org.uk

www.standingtogether.org.uk

www.idas.org.uk

How useful do you feel they would be? Could the advice be improved and has pregnancy been included in the advice?

This activity is based on your own research and application to your area of practice. There is no outline answer at the end of the chapter.

For midwives personally affected by domestic abuse

This chapter has alluded to the fact that your own life's experiences will inform how you practise in many respects. Unlike some personal issues the complexities of domestic abuse may mean that it may not be shared with colleagues. Please remember to care for your own physical and mental wellbeing and perhaps the helpline will provide you with the assistance and advice suited to you.

The 24-hour National Domestic Violence Freephone Helpline number is 0808 2000 247. The Helpline can give support, help and information over the telephone, wherever the caller might be in the country. The Helpline is staffed 24 hours a day by fully trained female helpline support workers and volunteers. All calls are completely confidential. Translation facilities for callers whose first language is not English and a service for callers who are deaf or hard of hearing are available.

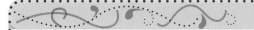

Chapter summary

This chapter has discussed the issue of domestic abuse during pregnancy and the role of the midwife in addressing this.

Addressing this topic is complicated by the midwife's own experiences and understanding of this type of abuse. It is vital that midwives are able to explore their own levels of empowerment and ability to use complex communication skills. Once you have established how and when you ask questions, the decision of how to proceed effectively is often the most challenging, and will be different in every case; this is where the ability to understand the woman's view of the situation is invaluable. You have been able to apply a model of change to the situation of abuse, thus helping you with framing your questioning. It has been noted within this chapter that child protection remains paramount in every case. Creating a safety plan with the woman may be the only contribution you have to offer during your relationship with her; however this should not be underestimated as it may in fact be lifesaving.

Midwives have much to offer the wider communities dealing with domestic abuse; therefore you have been encouraged to join local networks in order that you can share your experience and expertise with other professionals.

Activities: brief outline answers

Activity 7.5 Evidence-based practice [page 128]

On a very basic level your table should include similar information to the one below; you should be able to continue to expand on this as you continue to develop your own knowledge and experience of domestic abuse. Remember not just to focus on physical abuse; develop an awareness that areas such as financial abuse are difficult to quantify. Women are often victims of poly-abuse.

Obstetric wellbeing	Social wellbeing	Health behaviour
Late booker DNA appointments Random admissions to A&E or maternity unit Repeated urine infection Miscarriage IUD	Limited interaction with health and social care professionals Limited friend or family contact	Smoker Use of drugs and/or alcohol Reluctance to access healthcare

Activity 7.8 Critical thinking [page 129]

Jenny could be in either the pre-contemplation or contemplation stage of this model of change. In order to establish this you may need to ask further questions after acknowledging that this is not an acceptable situation. Perhaps you could ask her how she feels about this happening to her and how would you like you to help her. Once you have established where her mindset is, you will be able to develop your actions thereafter; importantly where possible this should be woman-led.

Activity 7.10 Developing communication skills [page 131]

When discussing a safety plan you could consider three aspects, as suggested by the Department of Health (*Responding to Domestic Abuse: A Handbook for Health Professionals* [2005]): (1) Safety in the relationship; (2) Leaving in an emergency; and (3) Safety when a relationship is over. Each element discusses how to create a safe environment, what the woman may need such as bank details, birth certificates, toys for the children and things for herself. Then finally, how to seek help and from whom during each period of time.

Further reading

Department of Health (2005) *Responding to Domestic Abuse: A Handbook for Health Professionals.* London: DH.

Harne, L. and Radford, J. (2008) *Tackling Domestic Violence: Theories, Policies and Practice.* Berkshire: Open University Press.

Useful websites

www.womensaid.org.uk

www.ncdv.org.uk

http://refuge.org.uk

www.standingtogether.org.uk

www.idas.org.uk

www.nhs.uk/Conditions/pregnancy-and-baby/pages/domestic-abuse-pregnant.aspx#close

Chapter 8
Substance misuse and pregnancy

Heather Passmore

NMC Standards for Pre-registration Midwifery Education

This chapter will address the following competencies:

Domain: Effective midwifery practice

Determine and provide programmes of care and support for women which:

- are made in partnership with women;
- involve other healthcare professionals when this will improve health outcomes.

Work in partnership with women and other care providers during the postnatal period to provide seamless care and interventions which:

- are appropriate to the woman's assessed needs, context and culture;
- draw in the skills of others to optimise health outcomes and resource use.

Contribute to enhancing the health and social wellbeing of individuals and their communities:

- planning and offering midwifery care within the context of public health policies.

Domain: Professional and ethical practice

Practise in accordance with relevant legislation:

- managing the complexities arising from ethical and legal dilemmas.

Maintain confidentiality of information:

- ensuring the confidentiality and security of written and verbal information acquired in a professional capacity;
- disclosing information about individuals and organisations only to those who have a right and need to know this information, and only once proof of identity and right to disclosure has been obtained.

Domain: Developing the individual midwife and others

Demonstrate effective working across professional boundaries and develop professional networks.

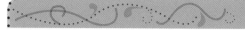

NMC Essential Skills Clusters

This chapter will address the following ESCs:

Cluster: Communication

3. Enable women to make choices about their care by informing women of the choices available to them and providing evidence-based information about benefits and risks of options so that women can make a fully informed decision.

- provides accurate, truthful and balanced information that is presented in such a way as to make it easily understood;
- respects women's autonomy when making a decision, even where a particular choice my result in harm to themselves or their unborn child, unless a court of law orders to the contrary.

8. Be confident in their own role within a multidisciplinary/multi-agency team.

- consults and explores solutions and ideas appropriately with others to enhance care;
- works inter-professionally as a means of achieving optimum outcomes for women.

Chapter aims

After reading this chapter you will be able to:

- consider ways of communicating with women who misuse substances to help them engage with service provision;
- discuss the impact of smoking and alcohol as legal substances that may adversely impact on health in pregnancy and for the child;
- identify the range of illegal substances that could be used and their possible effects on pregnancy and the baby;
- review how multidisciplinary and multi-agency working contributes to health promotion for women who misuse substances during pregnancy.

Introduction

The various forms of substance misuse that can impact on pregnancy and childbearing include smoking, alcohol and drugs. While some of these substances are legal and may be prescribed or bought over the counter, this does not necessarily confer safety to the mother or child. The impact on the woman and her family will be considered with particular reference to the sociological and psychological impact and concerns raised regarding possible safeguarding of the child. Midwives may care for women from a wide range of social backgrounds who may have a dependency on a substance[s] that could be detrimental both to them and to their unborn child, but each midwife must remain non-judgemental and supportive to the mother and her child.

There are women who smoke, drink and misuse drugs, but continue to be in employment while others have low self-esteem, disordered lifestyles and encounter many physical, social and psychological consequences of substance misuse. Midwives work with women from a variety of backgrounds, offer health promotion, care adequately for the woman and safeguard the baby/children. Multi agency involvement will be necessary to secure the best outcomes for the mother and her family.

All women should receive information on the effects of smoking, alcohol and drug use in pregnancy. While women may be concerned about the use of a substance prior to conception they can usually be advised that this is not likely to harm the baby. Within the first trimester, during the embryonic period the teratogenic effects that can result in malformation are the main concern. In the second and third trimesters, substance misuse is more likely to be associated with growth and functional impairment (Siney, 1999). Impaired placental function and fetal growth can result in a low birth weight baby, while chaotic drug use may result in preterm labour. The risk of sudden infant death is increased and babies may experience Neonatal Abstinence Syndrome when their mothers have been on certain drugs (Whittaker, 2003). While promoting a woman-centred approach to care, midwives should be mindful that women may feel worried and guilty about the effects of their substance misuse on the baby and as a consequence appear reluctant to admit to and discuss these issues (Klee *et al.*, 2002).

NHS values

It is of paramount importance that midwives practise in accordance with the NHS Values and Practice (Department of Health [DH], 2013a). The midwife should remain mindful that everyone counts irrespective of their behaviour and background. The value of working together for patients is pertinent and reflects the model of salutogenesis in that the journey through childbirth may enable a midwife to utilise her knowledge and skills, in combination with other health professionals and agencies, to support a woman to better health. This may improve the lives of the mother, her baby and other family members. All women should be treated with compassion as well as dignity and respect, irrespective of their life choices. Midwives should try to understand their priorities, needs, strengths and weakness and afford a level of communication which women understand and feel engaged, so remaining partners in their care.

Midwives have public health roles in particular for health improvement to help people live healthy lifestyles, make healthy choices and reduce health inequalities. This may be achieved by utilising their knowledge and skills to maximise their role in health and wellbeing through making every contact count. The National Institute for Health and Care Excellence (NICE) supports the delivery of the best possible care based on the best possible evidence and there are specific sources of evidence to support a reduction in the use of harmful substances during pregnancy, for example, PH26 Quitting smoking in pregnancy and following childbirth (NICE, 2010b) and NICE clinical guidance 110 – pregnancy and complex social factors (NICE, 2010a).

> ## Activity 8.1   *Reflection*
>
> The relationship between mother and midwife involves trust; consider how you facilitate women feeling able to answer questions at booking on social aspects of their life that involves behaviours that may be detrimental to their own health or that of the fetus/baby? Discuss what you would do with other midwives/students to compare the similarity and differences in your approach and responses. If they are different, consider why and perhaps you should try something different in practice and reflect on the process.
>
> *The answers to this activity will depend on your own reflections and experience.*

Providing information on these topics and then inviting women to share any concerns they have on these issues may enable women to be more forthcoming on their behaviours than direct questioning, which can make them feel as though they are being judged. Midwives act by being with women to promote the best outcomes for mother and baby.

Pre-conception substance management

To reduce any potential impact of substances such as smoking, alcohol and drugs, both women and men should be advised to stop or minimise their consumption at least three months prior to conception. Some evidence exists to support a decline in fertility due to smoking and alcohol adversely affecting spermatogenesis (Künzle *et al.*, 2002; Goverde *et al.*, 1995).

Management of prescribed medicines

Women with long-term conditions such as epilepsy or diabetes mellitus, or who take prescribed medicines, should be advised to consult with a GP/consultant to ensure they are on the lowest dosage of prescribed medication to maintain control of their condition or are prescribed an alternative drug with no known teratogenic effects on the baby. Good advice to offer women about over-the-counter medication such as paracetamol or ibuprofen is to use as few of these as possible. Women should be advised to check with their doctor, midwife or pharmacist whether a medicine is safe in pregnancy and to advise health professionals, such as dentists, that they are pregnant prior to treatment or any prescription.

Smoking

In 2014, 11.5% of pregnant women were known to be smokers at the time of delivery, and this figure demonstrates a fall from previous years. However statistics show huge variation across England, with the highest rate of smokers residing in the north of England and rates varying within cities with many women starting to smoke in adolescence (HSCIC, 2014a). This figure however might be misleadingly low as women try to conceal a behaviour on which they feel they may be adversely judged. While many women know of the harmful effects of smoking, nicotine is addictive and becoming pregnant does not always result in behaviour change (Prochaska, 1992). Teenagers are almost six times as likely to smoke throughout pregnancy as women who are over 35 (HSCIC, Infant Feeding Survey, 2010).

The major components causing adverse effects on health from smoking are nicotine and carbon monoxide, and also cyanide, which can interfere with cell development; however the smoke from tobacco contains at least 60 carcinogens. Nicotine is a stimulant and creates a feeling of euphoria. It is also addictive, the feelings being felt rapidly after inhaling. Nicotine has a half-life of 2–2.5 hours with a 75% decrease in nicotine levels after the last cigarette. Withdrawal signs and symptoms peak within 24–36 hours lasting for 10 days, though cravings can persist for months. Carbon monoxide and cyanide reduce the blood flow and bind with haemoglobin reducing the availability of oxygen to the fetus (Ashmead, 2003; Whittaker, 2003). To compensate, the fetal heart rate is raised after a cigarette is smoked.

The harmful effects of smoking during pregnancy have been well-documented (Eastham and Gosakan, 2010; BMA, 2004). Environmental smoke is associated with low birth weight, small for gestational age babies and sudden infant death. Public health action to reduce the impact of environmental smoke by, for example, the banning of smoking in public places may reduce these adverse consequences. Smoking cessation interventions in pregnancy have been shown to reduce the proportion of women who continue to smoke in late pregnancy, therefore reducing the consequences of this behaviour (Lumley *et al.*, 2009). Midwives and other health professionals should take responsibility to identify women who smoke in pregnancy and refer to smoking cessation services (see flow chart in NICE, 2010b), and advise them of the possible effects listed in Figure 8.1.

Activity 8.2   *Research and evidence-based practice*

Look up NICE Guidance (2010b) PH 26 Quitting smoking in pregnancy and following childbirth (**www.nice.org.uk/guidance/ph26/chapter/2-public-health-need-and-practice**) to determine the health risks of smoking in pregnancy.

- From the information you have read, which women are most likely to be smokers and with what effect?

- What strategies are suggested to help pregnant woman stop smoking?

- Look at the flow chart in this guidance for referral to smoking cessation services – do you know the points of contacts and how to communicate with them in your own area of practice?

An outline answer to this activity is given at the end of the chapter.

- Low birth weight babies (increased by about 40% – greater than that caused by heroin).
- Sudden infant death syndrome (risk tripled, BMA, 2004).
- Miscarriage.
- Preterm delivery.
- Intrauterine growth retardation (IUGR).
- Placental abruption.
- Stillbirth.
- Risk of infant mortality by an estimated 40% (DH, 2007).
- Babies of heavy smokers may be 'jittery'.
- Children of smokers suffer more respiratory infections.

Figure 8.1: Effects of tobacco on pregnancy and the neonate

Case study: Louise – smoking while pregnant

Louise, a 19-year-old gravida 2, attends for her booking appointment. When Amy, her midwife, asks whether she smokes Louise says yes, but she did this with her previous pregnancy and she doesn't want a big baby. She is smoking 10 cigarettes per day.

How might Amy provide advice to this woman?

In this case study, Louise has openly admitted that she smokes and can offer a reason for her behaviour. Amy needs to find ways of motivating Louise to quit smoking. She must explain that each pregnancy is different and the effects of smoking, while not evident with her first pregnancy, may present problems for her second pregnancy, and also affect the health of her first child. Amy will explain to Louise that should she go into preterm labour and have intrauterine growth retardation, and as both conditions are associated with smoking, the wellbeing of the baby may be compromised. Her existing child may also suffer the effects of passive smoking.

Some women find it difficult to say that they smoke because the pressure not to smoke during pregnancy is so intense. This, in turn, makes it difficult to ensure they are offered appropriate support. A carbon monoxide (CO) breath test is an immediate and non-invasive biochemical method for helping to assess whether or not someone smokes or is exposed to smoke. However, it is unclear as to what constitutes the best cut-off point for determining smoking status. Some suggest a CO level as low as three parts per million (ppm), others use a cut-off point of 6–10 ppm (NICE, 2010b). When trying to identify pregnant women who smoke, it is best to use a low cut-off point to avoid missing someone who may need help to quit.

Brief interventions involve opportunistic advice, discussion, negotiation or encouragement. They are commonly used in many areas of health promotion, and are delivered by a range of primary and community care professionals. While NICE (2010b) suggests that brief intervention therapy is not performed by midwives (remaining in the domain of NHS Stop Smoking services or equivalent), an established relationship can provide valuable opportunities for support.

The interventions vary from basic advice to more extended, individually focused attempts to identify and change factors that influence behaviour.

The primary goal of a brief intervention is to help the patient understand:

- what the consequences of their behaviour are likely to be;
- what they can do about it;
- what help is available.

Aveyard *et al.* (2005) and Ashmead (2003) suggests the use of a 10-minute conversation using the '5 As' model. These are listed below with suggested actions that Amy may use when caring for Louise.

1. **Ask:** at booking (and each antenatal visit), to identify how many cigarettes Louise is smoking and how frequently. Amy may ask what would be her top five reasons to stop smoking.

2. **Advise:** inform of the benefits of quitting; make the approach personalised. If Louise's partner smokes, could they both try and quit simultaneously?

3. **Assess:** Louise has indicated she is likely to continue to smoke in order to have a small baby. However, following advice she indicates she is willing to stop. Amy can offer support to help her to identify potential triggers, such as her partner smoking, or any stress.

4. **Assist:** Amy can make a referral to smoking cessation services. Louise will be advised to quit smoking and counselling offered to support this. If smoking cessation has not been successful she may be prescribed 2 weeks of nicotine replacement therapy (NRT) for use from the day she agrees to stop. Subsequent prescriptions will be issued on re-assessment (CO testing), providing she is still not smoking. Nicotine patches are the only form of NRT used during pregnancy (which should be removed before going to bed). Neither varenicline or bupropion should be offered to pregnant or breastfeeding women (NICE, 2010b).

5. **Arrange:** follow up with both Amy and smoking cessation services, with good documentation of action to support continuity of care and successful quitting. Support can be arranged for partners/family members, with information given on the danger of second-hand smoke. Relatives and friends should take care not to smoke around Louise or her existing child.

Case study: Outcome for Louise

At Louise's later antenatal visits, her CO breath test indicated a level of 12 ppm. While this level could be in part affected by NRT, Louise admitted that it was not working for her and she had resumed smoking. In addition her partner smoked and this could be adding to the level of smoke inhaled, causing an increase in CO level. No further NRT was therefore prescribed. Brief interventions alone are unlikely to be sufficient for Louise and so she should be provided with intensive and ongoing support throughout pregnancy and beyond. Amy should refer Louise to smoking cessation services and as well as regular appointments, with continuity of care, there will be regular monitoring of her smoking status using CO tests. The latter may encourage her to try to quit, and can also be a useful way of providing positive feedback if she tries to quit again.

What does NRT do?

NRT works by releasing nicotine steadily into the bloodstream at much lower levels than in a cigarette, which helps to control cravings without the tar, carbon monoxide and other poisonous chemicals present in tobacco smoke. The risks of nicotine are far outweighed by the risks of continuing to smoke. NRT should not be used while pregnant women are still smoking, as this would increase the amount of nicotine being passed to the fetus. Rather, NRT should be pre-scribed for use once the woman has already stopped smoking, or from the date she set to quit. The method of NRT (e.g. patches, gum, nasal spray, lozenges), which may produce some side effects, will be discussed to find the most suitable form related to previous smoking patterns.

Interventions to promote smoking cessation in pregnancy may include:

- Assessment of the woman's readiness to change (see below).
- Provision of advice and counselling (written and electronic resources and telephone support; cognitive behavioural therapy and motivational interviewing).
- Feedback of fetal wellbeing or CO measurement at each antenatal visit.
- NRT.
- Social support and encouragement – for example sessions in a non-clinical setting with other pregnant smokers who understood difficulties in quitting (Wilson, 2010).
- Other interventions such as hypnosis.

A Cochrane review of 72 trials concluded that smoking cessation interventions in pregnancy reduced the proportion of women who continued to smoke in late pregnancy and reduce low birth weight and preterm birth; therefore smoking cessation interventions should be available in all maternity care settings (Lumley *et al.*, 2009), however this is questioned in NICE (2010b). Chamberlain *et al.* (2013) indicate that psychosocial interventions such as providing incentives and counselling are of more benefit than health education on its own and there is no observed benefit in increasing the frequency or duration of the intervention.

A popular approach to explain behaviour change is that of Prochaska and DiClemente (1986). This 5-stage cycle, using a transtheoretical approach allows individuals to move backwards and forwards through the stages, according to the congruence of the advice given from the midwife and the stage of the individual. The skill of the midwife is to develop a behavioural understanding of the reasons for and against smoking to enable more effective interventions to be supported.

1. **Pre-contemplation:** not interested or given it any serious thought.
2. **Contemplation:** thinking about giving up, needs some help, advice, encouragement to make plans.
3. **Preparation:** deciding when and how to give up. The midwife can help plan a quit date and strategies for maximum support.
4. **Action:** trying to stop smoking so the midwife can help identify vulnerable situations and strategies to deal with these.
5. **Maintenance:** maintained cessation but still needs support.

To use this model efficiently, the midwife must communicate effectively and empathetically with the woman to determine which stage the woman has reached and her current feelings and experiences.

Electronic cigarettes, or e-cigarettes, are electrical devices that mimic real cigarettes but using an electronic cigarette or 'vaping' produces a vapour that is potentially less harmful than tobacco smoke. Many e-cigarettes contain nicotine, in unknown quantities, which may continue to be harmful in pregnancy. Currently there is no evidence of their ability to help people stop smoking. There are clinical trials in progress to test the quality, safety and effectiveness of e-cigarettes, but until these are complete, the government can't give any advice on them or recommend their use. A midwife would need reliable evidence before advising women on the safety of electronic cigarettes in pregnancy.

Smoking cessation services should be sensitive to the difficult circumstances many women who smoke find themselves in. They should take into account other socio-demographic factors such as age and ethnicity and ensure provision is culturally relevant, including provision for non-English speakers to access and use interpreting services. Difficulty in accessing services and concerns about being stigmatised may prevent women from attending stop smoking services; however involvement in the planning and development of these services may help to make them more accessible. Working in partnership with other agencies will increase awareness of stop smoking services and may increase referral rates for disadvantaged pregnant women. These agencies include substance misuse services, youth and teenage pregnancy support and mental health services. A midwives' toolkit is available to support women to stop smoking (**www.smokefree.nhs.uk/extranet/resources**).

Alcohol

Controversy exists as to what constitutes a safe level of alcohol intake during pregnancy. NICE (2008) suggests a safe intake of 1–2 units once or twice a week, although avoidance while trying to conceive and in the first 3 months is recommended. Other bodies, such as the National Organisation for Fetal Alcohol Syndrome (NOFAS) and Royal College of Midwives, recommend a zero intake to prevent any teratogenic effects of alcohol intake (NOFAS, 2011). Women may present at their booking interview concerned that they have been drinking, not realising they are pregnant. The midwife can provide reassurance that this is unlikely to have done harm; however further information on what constitutes a safe intake during pregnancy should be offered. The correlation between fetal alcohol syndrome and the amount of alcohol consumed in pregnancy is poor, with only one in 20 heavy drinkers delivering affected babies with fetal alcohol spectrum disorder, and as many drinkers also smoke it may be difficult to differentiate the main cause of intrauterine growth restriction (Prentice, 2010).

The analysis of the National Psychiatric Morbidity Survey 2007 showed that around 79,000 babies under 1 year were living with a parent who was classified as a 'hazardous or harmful' drinker (see Table 2 in this survey) which equates to 93,500 babies in the UK. Around 26,000 babies under 1 year are living with a parent who would be classed as a 'dependent' drinker. This equates to 31,000 babies in the UK (Manning, 2011).

In pregnancy, alcohol passes transplacentally to the fetus, which can adversely affect development and increase the risk of miscarriage (Kesmodel, 2002). Research by Harvard University on the developing brain indicates that 80% of brain cell development takes place by age three (Marmot, 2010). The brain appears particularly susceptible to the effects of alcohol. The ratio of white and grey matter can be altered, the nerve synapses and chemical neurotransmitters are affected and certain structures, for example the corpus callosum may be adversely affected. Fetal Alcohol Spectrum Disorder (FASD) is a series of preventable birth defects that can often go unrecognised or be misdiagnosed as autism or ADHD.

Fetal Alcohol Spectrum Disorder is an umbrella term that covers:

- fetal alcohol syndrome (FAS);
- alcohol related neurodevelopmental disorder;
- alcohol related birth defects;
- fetal alcohol effects;
- partial FAS.

(NOFAS, 2011)

- Facial anomalies – flat philtrum, thin upper lip, mid face hypoplasia, flat nasal bridge, short palpebral fissures.
- Central nervous system abnormalities, e,g. microcephaly, agenesis of corpus callosum, cerebellar hypoplasia.
- Neurodevelopmental abnormalities (reduced IQ, poor fine motor skills, behavioural problems).
- Intrauterine growth restriction and postnatal growth deficiency.

Table 8.1: Characteristic features of FAS

Some of the effects included within FASD can be associated with women who drank at some time in their pregnancy. While these effects attributed to alcohol are still more common in heavier drinkers, the problems also seem to happen at much lower drinking levels than for FAS. These lifelong disabilities are preventable and while freedom of choice remains a woman's prerogative, a clearer, consistent message of abstinence from alcohol in pregnancy may contribute to the reduction in FASD.

Activity 8.3   *Research and reflection*

Access the NOFAS website and watch the 26-minute file 'No alcohol, no risk' (**www. nofas-uk.org/database/videopage.php**), then reflect on the following questions:

- Has the film made you review how you provide information to mothers about alcohol intake in pregnancy?
- What information would you wish to record in the mother's notes on this issue?

- Devise several cue questions that you can use during antenatal visits to explore women's drinking patterns. Consider how this will enable you to ask the same thing more than once, in a slightly different way.
- How can a clear consistent message be offered to pregnant women on this topic?

The issues raised by this activity are discussed in the text below.

All pregnant women should be asked about their alcohol intake in pregnancy. The following questions are useful to assess a woman's level of alcohol dependency:

1. How much do you drink? (enquiring about one day at a time for the last week may be helpful).

2. How often do you drink?

3. What do you drink?

4. Do you take any other drugs/substances when you drink?

5. Do you have any medical conditions or take medicines that may be adversely affected by alcohol?

6. Are you or your family concerned about your drinking?

Reasons for concern should be further explored to determine need and strategies for change (Prentice, 2010).

The safe level of alcohol intake for pregnant women is nil; however for many women a small alcohol intake per week is acceptable. The volume of alcohol in a drink indicates the strength (alcohol by volume, ABV) and it is shown as a percentage on all bottles and cans. By knowing the alcoholic volume of a drink the number of units in the drink can be calculated. Midwives can show mothers how to calculate the number of units they are consuming.

$$\frac{\text{No. mL in the drink} \times \text{strength (ABV) on the label}}{1000} = \text{No. units in drink}$$

e.g. A bottle of wine

$$\frac{750 \text{ mL} \times 13\%}{1000} = 9.75$$

175 mL glass of wine (13% ABV) is 2.28 units.

A large glass of wine = 250 mL (third of a bottle); a medium glass is 175 mL; a small glass is 125 mL.

A review of the above formula indicates how care must be taken with tables, e.g. Table 8.2, that state the alcohol by volume per glass, with no indication of strength or glass size.

	Units
Single measure of whisky	1
Glass of wine	2
Pint of beer or lager	2
Bottle of alcopops	1.5

Table 8.2: What is in a unit of alcohol?

Activity 8.4   *Critical thinking*

While you are taking a booking history, the woman tells you that she drinks a glass of wine 3 days a week after work and enjoys a couple of pints of cider (5% ABV) at the weekend.

How many units is she consuming per week?

What advice would you give this woman?

An answer to this activity is given at the end of the chapter.

Case study: Giving advice on alcohol intake

Justine, a 38-year-old primigravida attends for her booking interview at 10 weeks' gestation. She works as a director for a marketing firm. Satya, her midwife, asks about her alcohol intake. Justine replies that she attends a lot of functions and often has a drink most evenings to relax. She goes on to say that she has cut down her consumption of alcohol since she realised she was pregnant.

Satya uses the Alcohol Use Disorders Identification Test (AUDIT), a well-validated tool developed by the World Health Association (Babor et al., 2001) to determine Justine's level of risk from alcohol use.

Risk level	Score	Action
Low risk	0–7	Positive reinforcement
Hazardous	8–15	Brief intervention
Harmful	16–19	Extended brief intervention
Possible dependence	20–40	Further assessment

Justine has a score of 14.

Alternatively Satya could have used the FAST Alcohol Screening Test, a four-item initial screening test taken from AUDIT (PHE, 2013a). It was developed for busy clinical settings as a two-stage initial screening test that is quick to administer since more than 50% of patients are identified by using just the first question – How often have you had six or more units (as female), on a single occasion in the last year?

If Justine's level of drinking was higher, NOFAS (2011) suggests the use of two other tools: the T-ACE (tolerance–annoyance, cut down and eye-opener) alcohol screening questionnaire where behaviour may be affected by alcohol and the TWEAK (tolerance, worried, eye-opener, amnesia and cut down) questionnaire for people with high levels of binge drinking.

Satya thinks carefully about how she might most effectively support Justine. She decides to use a brief intervention strategy using the acronym FRAMES (PHE, 2013b) as this is a useful health promotion intervention for someone with high self-efficacy.

- ***F**eedback, personalised to express concern over alcohol intake and assess understanding.*

- ***R**esponsibility, determine with the woman her level of concern.*

- ***A**dvice, offered in a clear and practical way.*

- ***M**enu, providing a variety of options.*

- ***E**mpathy, the use of warm, reflective statements to indicate that the woman may be surprised by the new knowledge she is gaining and that it does not reflect badly on her.*

- ***S**elf-efficacy, boosting confidence to recognise previous success in changing behaviour.*

The advice Satya gives to Justine is based on NICE guidance (NICE, 2008).

- *As she is 10 weeks' pregnant she should stop drinking until the first three months of pregnancy are complete to avoid an increased risk of miscarriage.*

- *Justine should drink no more than 1–2 units of alcohol once or twice a week. There is uncertainty about how much alcohol is safe to drink in pregnancy, but at this low level there is no evidence of harm to the unborn baby.*

- *Satya explains that Justine should not get drunk or binge drink (more than 7.5 UK units of alcohol on a single occasion) because this can harm her unborn baby.*

- *To avoid all possible alcohol-related risks, Satya encourages Justine to avoid drinking any alcohol while she is pregnant.*

On realising the risks and with support from Satya, Justine reduced her alcohol intake to one large glass of wine at the end of the week.

Illegal drug use in pregnancy

Many pregnant women who use illegal substances may not access antenatal and other healthcare services, due to complex social factors, including:

- Feeling overwhelmed by the involvement of multiple agencies.

- Being unfamiliar with antenatal care services.

- Practical problems that make it difficult for them to attend antenatal appointments, such as no transport or costs of transport.

- Difficulty in communicating with healthcare staff, 'feeling they don't speak the right language and won't be understood'.

- Anxiety about the attitudes of healthcare staff with fear of being judged.

(NICE, 2010a)

Based on the prevalence of illicit drug use some women may be using illegal substances without the knowledge of the midwife or other health and social care services.

Research summary: Prevalence of illicit drug use

Around 1 in 11 (8.8%) adults aged 16–59 had taken an illicit drug in 2013–2014; however this proportion was doubled in the 16–24 age group (18.9%). The levels of drug use were marginally higher than the previous year, though significantly lower than in 1996. The use of cocaine, ecstasy, LSD and heroin increased (ONS, 2014). Frequent drug use is defined as 'those that have taken any illicit drug more than once a month on average in the last year' (ONS, 2014, Section 3.3).

A pregnant woman who misuses substances (alcohol and/or drugs) needs supportive and coordinated care during pregnancy if she is not to feel overwhelmed by interactions with too many different agencies. This may be helped by the following:

- A single coordinated care plan jointly developed across agencies including information about opiate replacement therapy in care plans.

- Information of why and when information about them will be shared with other agencies, for example on progress made and current therapy or accommodation situation.

- The services she uses should ideally be accessible at one site – for example, a Children's Centre.

- Care from a named midwife who has specialised knowledge and experience in caring for pregnant women who misuse substances. A direct telephone number for this named midwife should be made available. This midwife can signpost to other services.

- Text messaging may assist in providing a reminder for appointments and the midwife may investigate support for transportation to antenatal checks.

(NICE, 2010a)

The analysis of the National Psychiatric Morbidity Survey 2007 showed that around 43,000 babies under 1 year were living with a parent who has used an illegal drug in the past year, equivalent to 51,000 babies across the UK. Around 16,500 babies under 1 year are living with a parent who has used Class A drugs in the past year, equivalent to 19,500 babies in the UK (Manning, 2011).

Case study: Postnatal care for a drug user

Angie, a community midwife, visits Ailsa who is 2 days postnatal at home for the first time. The room is quite dark and there is a smell in the room that Angie can't quite identify. There are several men in the house and she is unsure who is the baby's father. Angie notices some fizzy drink cans that are partly crushed lying on the coffee table with some matches.

- *What intuitive knowledge might Angie use in this situation?*
- *How might she communicate with Ailsa to try to understand her social situation?*
- *How important is it for Angie to know what substances Ailsa may be taking?*
- *What is the relevance of being unsure of who the father may be?*

The midwife has a responsibility to safeguard the baby, so Angie will need to make a referral to her local safeguarding team. However, she should inform Ailsa of this action. She needs to complete a Common Assessment Framework (CAF) form to support this referral. Knowledge of what substances are being taken may enable the midwife, in conjunction with other professionals, to determine possible risks to the mother and her baby (see Table 8.3). Angie should also consider who the father of the child is and whether, in the above circumstance, there may be any risk of domestic abuse or sexual exploitation requiring protection to be initiated for the mother as well as the baby.

What is a Common Assessment Framework (CAF) form?

A CAF form is a standard, nationally available tool to determine whether a child has unmet needs. It was developed by the Department for Children, Schools and Families (DCSF) in association with national children's charities. Many authorities have their own guidelines on using the form. See for example, the guidelines from the Bury Council website: **www.bury.gov.uk/index.aspx?articleid=3370**

The Centre for Maternal and Child Enquiries, in its discussion on maternal deaths where substance misuse has made a significant contribution to the cause of deaths (CMACE, 2011), supports the need for information sharing. These women may conceal or minimise the nature and extent of their substance misuse, fearing a judgemental attitude and child protection involvement.

Substance [Class]	Street names	Taken as	General effects include	Effects on fetus/neonate
Cannabis [B]	Grass, Pot, Skunk, Dope, Blow, Weed, Wacky, Backy, Puff	Smoked in rolled up cigarette papers Baked in cakes Drunk in tea	Mild sedative/hallucinogen Relaxed, talkative, giggly, hungry Anxiety, panic attacks, bloodshot eyes, poor balance Lung, mouth, throat cancer, chest infections	Uncertain and may be associated with effects of smoking and/or alcohol use
Cocaine [A] (Crystal Meth is similar, but effects last longer)	Coke, Freebase, Nose Candy, Stones, Blow, Rocks, Snow	Inhaled (snorted) Injected or swallowed Heated and smoked in pipe or tin foil	CNS stimulant giving a quick high lasting 15–30 minutes; highly addictive Depression – coming down from high ('crashing'). Muscle twitches, severe tremors, violent behaviour, hallucinations, insomnia	Can cause miscarriage, placental abruption, intrauterine growth restriction, intrauterine death and stillbirth, low birth weight babies, preterm birth, underdevelopment of organs and/or limbs Use in pregnancy can result in vascular compromise within the fetal central nervous system causing jitteriness, irritability, hypotonia, poor feeding, abnormal sleep pattern
Ecstasy [A]	MDMA, MDA, MBDB, 'E'	Swallowed in tablet form May be mixed with other substances	Euphoria, confident, energised, chatty Confusion, dilated pupils, hallucinations, paranoia Dehydration, raised body temperature, raised pulse Oliguria, kidney damage, heart disease, liver damage, depression	No conclusive evidence of effects on pregnancy however users may have poor physical and mental health
Heroin [A]	Brown, Skag, H, Horse, Gear, Smack	Injected Smoked in a pipe Snorted as a powder	Amenorrhoea, malnutrition, anaemia and vitamin deficiencies Risks of IV drug use – hepatitis and HIV infection	May cause abruption placenta or placenta praevia, gestational hypertension, breech presentation, multiple births, preterm labour, small for dates babies

Drug	Names	Route	Effects	Effects in pregnancy
Ketamine [C]	Special K, Vitamin K, 'K', Green, Kit Kat, Super K	Inhaled (snorted) but can be swallowed or injected	Affects CNS, loss of sensation including pain and bladder control Hallucinations, flashbacks, depression, slurred speech, blackouts, panic attacks	Effects not clear. Although not specific to pregnancy, ketamine can cause bladder damage
Amphetamine [B]	Speed, Whizz	Swallowed	CNS stimulant Hypertension, tachycardia, hyperthermia Vascular and heart problems including strokes/heart attack	Heavy users may experience poor general health. Causes vasoconstriction and hypertension that may cause fetal hypoxia. May be associated with an increase in small for gestation age and preterm infants
Benzodiazepines Prescription only Medicine [C]	e.g. Valium, Temazepam	Orally	Depresses CNS Sudden withdrawal can result in severe anxiety symptoms, hallucinations and seizure	High doses may be associated with hypotonia, hypothermia, hyperbilirubinaemia, feeding difficulties with poor sucking, respiratory difficulties with apnoea Can delay the onset of neonatal abstinence syndrome if taken with opiates
LSD (Lysergic acid Diethylamide) [A]	Acid, Rainbows, Tripper, Micro Dot	Swallowed	Hallucinogenic, flashbacks, frightening, euphoria, self-harm, panic and confusion, mental health problems	No evidence of congenital malformations and no conclusive evidence of other risks in pregnancy

Table 8.3: Drugs and their effects

(Sources: **www.talktofrank.com**; Siney, 1999; Whittaker, 2003; White Ribbon Alliance – **www.white-ribbon.org.uk**)

> ## Activity 8.5   *Critical thinking*
>
> Consider whether a baby should remain with a mother who continues to use illegal substances. Refer to the NMC (2015) *Professional Standards of Practice and Behaviour for Nurses and Midwives* and local safeguarding procedures to help clarify your thoughts.
>
> Then discuss the question with your peers and mentors.
>
> Using the information in the 'Tools' section of NICE guidance on pregnancy in women with complex social factors (**www.nice.org.uk/guidance/cg110**) consider what is required by a midwife in terms of service organisation and training to meet the social and psychological needs of these women, and how care delivery will be enhanced, in order to fulfil the requirements of antenatal care within NICE guidance (**www.nice.org.uk/guidance/CG62**).
>
> Again, discuss your thoughts with your peers and mentors.
>
> *The answers to this activity will depend on your own thoughts and experience, so no outline answer is given.*

CMACE (2011, p139) states that women may conceal or minimise the nature and extent of their substance misuse, often fearing a censorious approach or child protection involvement. It is important that midwives are self-reflective and aware, in order to prevent this happening in their practice.

Early information sharing between the GP, maternity and addiction services is essential. Management should include drug-monitoring measures, such as regular urine screening, particularly where substitute prescribing is used.

> ### Case study: Reflections on a difficult situation
>
> *Franka is a 27-year-old gravida 3 whose previous two children have been placed in care as she has a history of drug and alcohol abuse. She was sexually abused as a child, and she has a history of heroin, cocaine and cannabis use and is now Hepatitis C positive. She is maintained on Subutex 4 mg. Both she and her partner have been imprisoned on several occasions for numerous crimes including theft, burglary, possessing an offensive weapon, criminal damage and soliciting for prostitution. They have been evicted from their bed and breakfast accommodation for non-payment of fees and the council are now not obliged to house them as it is considered they have made themselves homeless through this action.*
>
> - *What are the parameters for referral and to whom in the case of Franka?*
>
> *Franka booked at 18 weeks' pregnant saying she didn't realise she was pregnant. Her community midwife discussed her booking with the named midwife for substance misuse who became the lead carer. The consultant obstetrician and paediatrician were involved and delivery planned for hospital due to*

chaotic home circumstances and the possibility of neonatal abstinence syndrome. She involved the social worker and jointly a referral was made to the local Safeguarding Team and a case conference was convened. Engagement with services and different agencies is being monitored throughout her pregnancy. She is being induced at 38 weeks' pregnant, as the baby is small for gestational age. Following delivery she must stay in for 5 days as the baby is subject to an interim care order and review.

- What do you anticipate will be the outcome of the review and why?

Despite Franka showing an interest in breastfeeding once her baby was born, the baby showed signs of neonatal abstinence syndrome including a high pitched cry, hyperactivity and hypertonic movements, difficultly in settling after feeds, regurgitation and vomiting, hungry but poor feeding ability, temperature instability and increased heart rate requiring admission to the neonatal intensive care unit. Franka requested discharge from the postnatal ward but then visited her baby irregularly and was unable to establish breastfeeding. She and her partner were unable to secure suitable housing and a care order was placed on the child who was then fostered and was to be placed for adoption.

- What may be the impact of taking women to visit a neonatal intensive care unit if their babies are likely to require admission to the unit due to maternal substance misuse?

Outline answers to the questions in this case study are given at the end of the chapter.

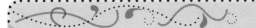

Chapter summary

Substance misuse in pregnancy is a key public health issue not only because of the impact on the fetus and the child, but because the harm is preventable. Midwives need to be non-judgemental, promote the NHS values and use a range of health promotion techniques to enable women to make healthy choices and take actions for harm reduction. Midwives should enable mothers to understand the consequences of their behaviour, what they can do about it and what help is available with support to access these services.

Not all substances that can be harmful during pregnancy are illegal. Midwives should be able to advise women about use of over-the-counter medications as well as offering support on quitting smoking and information about the dangers of smoking and drinking alcohol during pregnancy. It is important to make the point that the unborn baby will be at risk as well as the mother herself.

Women who use illegal drugs may have other psychological, social or health problems and midwives are likely to need to refer the woman to other agencies. In particular, if the welfare of a baby or other children is at risk, the midwife will need to make a referral to the local safeguarding team. Midwives need to complete a Common Assessment Framework (CAF) form to support this referral, and should also inform the woman concerned that they are doing this.

Activities: brief outline answers

Activity 8.2 Research and evidence-based practice [page 141]

All the available research (and there is a lot of it) tell us that smoking during pregnancy can cause serious pregnancy-related health problems. As well as the possibility of the baby being small at birth, women who smoke during pregnancy are more likely than those who don't to have a complicated labour or to lose their baby either early in the pregnancy (miscarriage), late in the pregnancy (resulting in a stillbirth) or in infancy.

Children who have been exposed to tobacco smoke in the womb because of their mother smoking are more likely to suffer from wheezy illnesses in childhood. Children growing up around smokers are also more likely to suffer from respiratory problems including asthma, bronchitis and pneumonia as well as problems of the ear, nose and throat.

There have also been research findings which suggest that poor levels of achievement in school and behaviour problems may be linked in some way to exposure to smoking in the womb.

Many mothers find it easier to give up smoking completely rather than cutting down, and giving up completely is the best course of action for your health and for your baby's health too. There is plenty of advice and support available to help you with this.

Answer is based on NICE Guidance (2010) PH 26 Quitting Smoking in Pregnancy and Following Childbirth (www. nice.org.uk/guidance/ph26/chapter/2-public-health-need-and-practice).

Activity 8.4 Critical thinking [page 148]

This woman is consuming per week 6 units from wine (though this does depend on the size of the glass) plus 4.5 units from cider.

She should be advised to cut out alcohol completely in the first trimester of pregnancy to be sure of avoiding FASD. In the second and third trimesters, consumption of alcohol is best avoided completely, although NICE (2008) suggests that 1–2 units per week will not be harmful.

Case study: Reflections on a difficult situation [page 154]

What are the parameters for referral and to whom in the case of Franka?

Both Franka and her baby will be considered in need of consultant obstetric and paediatric care with significant support and assessment from the local safeguarding team to determine suitability for the baby to remain in their care.

Franka will be referred to her local substance misuse midwife or vulnerable persons' team. If this doesn't include the midwife with responsibility for safeguarding, there should be an immediate referral. Social services should be informed to determine any possibility of securing housing for the family. Her GP should be contacted (if she is registered with one) to make them aware of her pregnancy plus the substance misuse service supplying her maintenance doses of Subutex. The neonatal intensive care unit should be involved to plan for care of the neonate with risk of neonatal abstinence syndrome.

What do you anticipate will be the outcome of the review and why?

The safety of the child is paramount and any decisions should be made in the best interests of the child. The ability of the parents to meet the basic needs of the baby will be considered. Evidence of neonatal abstinence syndrome plus other behaviours exhibited by Franka could suggest continued illegal drug use in addition to taking Subutex. These behaviours combined with being homeless were presented to the case review held immediately after birth, and the decision was made to remove the baby from the care of her mother with recommendation for adoption.

What may be the impact of taking women to visit a neonatal intensive care unit if their babies are likely to require admission to the unit due to maternal substance misuse?

It may be unsettling and anxiety provoking as the environment is strange, full of machines and equipment available to support life. This may make the woman feel guilty for her actions or it could make her want to 'run away' from the difficulties that her baby may face in the early days/weeks of its life. Staff involved in the care of the baby need to remain non-judgemental but aware of the outcomes of any safeguarding meetings and where possible involve the mother and father in the care provided to the baby.

Further reading

The following publications all give essential information:

NICE (2008) *Antenatal Care.* **www.nice.org.uk/guidance/CG62**

NICE (2010) *Quitting Smoking in Pregnancy and Following Childbirth.* Guidance (2010) PH 26 **www.nice.org.uk/guidance/ph26**

NICE (2010) *Pregnancy and Complex Social Factors.* NICE Clinical Guideline 110.

Whittaker, A. (2003) *Substance Misuse in Pregnancy: A Resource Pack for Professionals in Lothian.* Edinburgh: NHS Lothian.

Useful websites

www.alcohollearningcentre.org.uk
Public Health England Alcohol Learning Resources.

www.nta.nhs.uk/who-service.aspx
National Treatment Agency for Substance Misuse website.

www.talktofrank.com
An A–Z on drugs and their effects and where to find local support services.

www.white-ribbon.org.uk
The White Ribbon Alliance website. Provides educational resources on smoking, alcohol and illegal drugs – mainly for schools' use but helpful in other situations too.

Chapter 9
Promoting parenting in midwifery

Sam Chenery-Morris

NMC Standards for Pre-Registration Midwifery Education

This chapter will address the following competencies:

Domain: Effective midwifery practice:

Communicate effectively with women and their families throughout the pre-conception, antenatal, intrapartum and postnatal periods. Communication will include:

- listening to women and helping them to identify their feelings and anxieties about their pregnancies, the birth and the related changes to themselves and their lives;
- enabling women to think through their feelings;
- enabling women to make informed choices about their health and healthcare;
- actively encouraging women to think about their own health and the health of their babies and families, and how this can be improved;
- communicating with women throughout their pregnancy, labour and the period following birth.

Care for and monitor women during the puerperium, offering the necessary evidence-based advice and support regarding the baby and self-care. This will include:

- providing advice and support on feeding babies and teaching women about the importance of nutrition in child development;
- providing advice and support on hygiene, safety, protection, security and child development;
- enabling women to address issues about their own, their babies' and their families' health and social wellbeing;
- monitoring and supporting women who have postnatal depression or other mental illnesses;
- providing advice on bladder control;
- advising women on recuperation;
- providing advice on contraception;
- supporting women to care for ill/pre-term babies or those with disabilities.

Domain: Professional and ethical practice

Work collaboratively with the wider healthcare team and agencies in ways which:

- value their contribution to health and care;
- enable them to participate effectively in the care of women, babies and their families;
- acknowledge the nature of their work and the context in which it is placed.

The wider healthcare team and agencies will include those who work in:

- healthcare;
- social care;
- social security, benefits and housing;
- advice, guidance and counselling;
- child protection;
- the law.

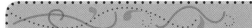

NMC Essential Skills Clusters

This chapter will address the following ESCs:

Cluster: Initial consultation between the woman and the midwife

Women can trust/expect a newly registered midwife to:

3. Work collaboratively with other healthcare professionals and external agencies.

Cluster: Normal labour and birth

6. Support women and their partners in the birth of their babies.
7. Facilitate the mother and baby to remain together.

Cluster: Initiation and continuance of breastfeeding

2. Respect social and cultural factors that may influence the decision to breastfeed.
4. Support women to breastfeed.
4. Recognise appropriate infant growth and development, including where referral for further advice/action is required.

Chapter aims

After reading this chapter you will be able to:

- understand how and where midwives can promote bonding and attachment in relation to the developing fetus during pregnancy and with the baby in the postnatal period with all women;
- recognise parents who require further support to enhance the start their baby has in life;
- consider strategies which promote optimal parenting.

Introduction

This chapter will consider how the midwife can promote parenting skills throughout the contact period with the woman and her family. Ideally the best start for any baby is a healthy woman and partner pre-conceptually, therefore factors which impact upon optimal fetal development will be covered. During the antenatal period the midwife can support the woman in her knowledge of fetal development. Increased knowledge of fetal stages of development such as hearing, movement and growth can be used to promote positive attachment and bonding to the unborn baby. In the antenatal period the midwife is assessing women and their family interactions to see who may require further support with parenting. Theories of attachment will be considered to help your ability to promote bonding antenatally and postnatally. The midwife's role in the postnatal period includes safety, feeding and caring for the neonate but also understanding and supporting positive early family interactions which promote childhood development.

Before conception

It might seem strange to start a chapter on parenting with pre-conceptual care, but there are behaviours that couples can alter which increase their chance of conception and a healthy baby. A healthy baby can reduce parenting stress, as this chapter will show. While pre-conceptual care is available on the NHS free of charge, few couples access this. The tests available to women, to assess their level of immunity and screen for infectious diseases are repeated in the early antenatal period, but having immunity or treatment for an infection prior to conception can prevent some problems for the baby. Similarly health lifestyles, such as smoking cessation, alcohol and drug abstinence and nutritional supplementation will prevent some fetal and lifelong problems.

Women and their partners can access pre-conceptual care and advice from a GP, midwife and some nurse practitioners or practice nurses, at their local surgery or family planning clinic.

The antenatal period

While following this advice pre-conceptually or in the antenatal period does not guarantee a baby will be born without health needs, it optimises its chances. Once a woman is pregnant, the midwife will reiterate these points to promote healthy fetal development. The antenatal period is also a time when the midwife identifies other risks which may impair a woman and her partner's parenting ability.

Concept summary: Sub-optimal parenting

It is known that factors which make parenting more difficult include:

- negative experiences of being parented;
- poverty, social deprivation and isolation, poor housing and environment;
- divorce, separation and lone parenting;
- culture of long working hours for men and women;
- young parental age.

Sub-optimal parenting impacts on outcomes (educational failure, criminality, antisocial behaviour, poor mental and physical health) that predispose to inequalities in the next generation.

Topic	Benefit/problem	Advice
Smoking	Smoking may make men and women less fertile. Smoking females are 3 to 4 times more likely than non-smokers to take longer than a year to conceive.	Cessation of maternal and partner's smoking (or cut down as much as possible)
		Support from smoking cessation counsellors.
	Smoking males have an average of 13–17% lower sperm counts than non-smokers, as well as having an increased number of abnormal sperm in their ejaculate.	Male fertility is affected by low zinc, selenium, vitamin C and alcohol, obesity and smoking.
	There are significant risks to the health, and life, of a baby if the mother smokes. These include the risk of miscarriage, premature birth and stillbirth, of placental abnormalities, low birth weight and, after birth, sudden infant deaths. It is estimated that about one third of all perinatal deaths in the UK are caused by smoking.	
Diet	Low folic acid levels known to increase chance of neural tube defects, including spina bifida.	Folic acid supplementation of 400 micrograms per day for most women until 12 weeks' gestation but 5 mg if previously affected by neural tube defects, diabetes or epilepsy.
	Low vitamin D can cause rickets in children.	Vitamin D supplementation
		Avoid certain foods – excess vitamin A.
	Salmonella.	Found in liver, unpasteurised cheeses, pâté, soft boiled eggs.
		Handwashing when touching raw meat products; heat ready-made meals thoroughly.

(Continued)

161

Table 9.1 (Continued)

Topic	Benefit/problem	Advice
	Listeriosis if caught in pregnancy can cause stillbirth or miscarriage.	– Do not eat unpasteurised goat's milk or their products. Women planning a pregnancy or who are pregnant should avoid soft ripened cheese like Camembert, Brie and blue vein type cheeses. Hard cheeses like Cheshire and Cheddar are fine. Listeria is frequently found in: – Cooked chilled meals – cook until piping hot – Ready to eat poultry – cook until piping hot – Pâté – Liver sausage – Soft whipped ice cream.
	Toxoplasmosis caught in pregnancy can cause miscarriage, still birth, blindness and brain damage.	Some simple advice to avoid Toxoplasmosis includes: – Do not eat raw or undercooked meat (Parma ham, salami etc.) – Wash hands after handling raw meat – Wash thoroughly all fruit, vegetables and salads to remove dirt – Wash hands after handling cats – Wear rubber gloves when changing cat litter trays, then wash gloves and hands – Wear gardening gloves when handling soil – Cover outdoor sandboxes.
	Caffeine intake above 200 mg is associated with low birth weight and sometimes miscarriage.	Reduce caffeine intake. New advice from the Food Standards Agency advises pregnant women to limit caffeine to less than 200 mg; the equivalent of 2 cups of coffee a day.

Alcohol	Risk of fetal alcohol syndrome. Alcohol affects male and female infertility and can contribute to miscarriage. Excessive alcohol consumption has also been linked to an early menopause in women.	Minimum alcohol intake, abstinence is best. There is no nationally accepted standard of what is considered a safe alcohol limit during pregnancy.
Drug misuse	This includes prescription drugs as well as illicit drugs. Some drugs have a teratogenic effect on the developing fetus; this may lead to a congenital malformation.	Discuss all drug use with your GP prior to conception; certain anti-epilepsy drugs are harmful, but safer preparations can be prescribed for conception. The use of illicit hard drugs such as heroin is clearly associated with abnormalities and dependency syndromes in babies. These drugs should be avoided at all costs.
Immunity	Risk of contracting rubella in pregnancy – severely affects fetal development, can cause blindness, deafness and developmental delay. Rubella infection in the first 8 to 10 weeks of pregnancy results in fetal damage in up to 90% of infants.	Check immunity (blood test) and immunise if not protected 1 month prior to pregnancy only – if already pregnant immunise postnatally.
Contact with animals	Certain animals can carry bacteria that can cause harm to a developing embryo. Cats may carry Toxoplasmosis. Sheep and goats may carry Brucella and chlamydiosis.	Basic hygiene is very important. Wear gloves if cleaning cat litter, handling animals or working in the garden, avoid contact with sheep during lambing. Always wash your hands thoroughly afterwards. If you work closely with animals or you have any specific worries your GP will discuss these with you.

Table 9.1: Antenatal and pre-conceptual advice

When the midwife has knowledge of each woman's social and familial circumstances, she will be able to promote parenting throughout the antenatal period. It is the first appointment, called the booking visit, where a midwife finds out about a woman's pregnancy, previous medical and obstetric history and social circumstances. This information is used to offer additional advice.

Activity 9.1 — *Decision-making*

With a colleague work out who you would refer the following women to:

1. A woman who says she smokes and would like help to reduce this.
2. A woman who has had previous anxiety which required treatment with medication.
3. A woman who is ambivalent about her pregnancy.
4. A 16-year-old who is pregnant.
5. A woman who discloses she abuses drugs or alcohol.

The answers to all but Case 3 are in the preceding chapters (see pages 140–141, 101–103, 44–45, 145–153) and not repeated at the end of this chapter. Case 3 will be discussed in the text that follows.

While undertaking this activity you may wonder why ambivalence to pregnancy matters. With contraceptive services widely available in the UK and access to abortion, you may not think that women would continue a pregnancy if they did not want to, or if they were undecided about it. Yet, the National Survey of sexual attitudes and lifestyles in the UK undertaken in 2013 revealed that 16.2% of pregnancies which resulted in a birth in the past year scored as unplanned, 29.0% as ambivalent and 54.8% as planned (Wellings *et al.*, 2013)

The problem with unplanned pregnancies is twofold: there can be negative effect on women's health and poorer outcome of pregnancies (Mohllajee *et al.*, 2007). Women whose pregnancy is unplanned usually present for antenatal care later, are more prone to antenatal and postnatal depression and relationship breakdowns. Their babies have lower birth weight, poorer mental and physical health during childhood and do less well with cognitive development (Wellings *et al.*, 2013). The reasons pregnancies are unplanned are strongly associated with the following: age of first sexual contact below 16 years; smoking; recent use of drugs (not cannabis) and lower educational attainment (Wellings *et al.*, 2013).

Pregnancy intention can be measured in several ways. Mohllajee *et al.* (2007) used intended, unwanted, mistimed or ambivalent; they found unwanted and ambivalent pregnancies tend to have poorer outcomes than planned or mistimed. The Millennium Cohort study (Carson *et al.*, 2013) used the terms unplanned (and unhappy); mistimed (unplanned but happy); planned and then broke this down further into time to conception (under 12 months; over 12 months; received ovulation treatment and received artificial reproductive technologies). Their research concluded that mistimed and unplanned pregnancies resulted in children who exhibited more behavioural difficulties than those whose pregnancy was planned.

In relation to planning and providing midwifery care and in promoting positive parenting it is appropriate to ask women how they feel about their current pregnancy so those with ambivalence can be offered more structured preparation for parenthood classes to try to reduce their child's inequality later in life. Clearly if a pregnancy is unplanned and the parents are teenagers, they have not finished their own education, have limited income and are often living with their parents. Extra support, such as the Family Nurse Partnership which offers a structured programme of antenatal and postnatal motivational interviewing for two years, can help promote effective parent–child interactions and improve the quality of life for young parents as well.

The Child Health Promotion Programme (DH, 2008) uses two terms which classify prospective parents. These classifications are used to identify parents who may benefit from further support and services. The terms are universal and progressive. Universal is the term used for information, advice and services offered to all families whereas progressive is the term used for families who would benefit from additional services and support. In some areas of the UK the health visitor assesses families' needs; in other areas the midwife, as the first point of call, completes this assessment.

The early identification of families who may require extra support is based on evidence that links children's educational and social development to their start in life. For instance parents with few or no educational qualifications, poor employment prospects or mental health problems benefit from extra support to promote their child's social development and readiness for school so they can attain their educational potential. The evidence from the Social Exclusion Task Force (2007) shows a link between parental disadvantage and adverse children's outcomes. Families in need of progressive care are not always easy to identify but include:

- young parents;
- educational problems;
- parents not in education, employment or training;
- families living in poverty;
- families living in unsatisfactory accommodation;
- parents with mental problems;
- unstable partner relationships;
- intimate partner abuse;
- parents with a history of antisocial behaviour;
- families with low social capital;
- ambivalence about becoming a parent;
- stress in pregnancy;
- low self-esteem or resilience;
- a history of abuse, mental illness or alcoholism in mother's own family.

(DH, 2008)

Identifying families who would benefit from further support and care is only part of the booking interview. All pregnant women should receive the advice given in Table 9.2.

Timing	Opportunity/recommended care	Rationale
At the first contact with a healthcare professional	All the information in Table 9.1 above	To optimise the pregnancy outcome of a healthy baby
At booking (ideally by 10 weeks)	Discuss how the baby develops during pregnancy in conjunction with distribution of *The Pregnancy Book* (DH, 2009) to first time mothers	To inform parents of fetal development to promote attachment
	Offer nutritional and dietary advice, including vitamin D supplementation for women at risk of vitamin D deficiency	For optimal fetal development
	Offer details of the 'Healthy Start' programme (**www.healthystart.nhs.uk**) which includes benefits of breastfeeding, including workshops	To promote optimal infant feeding
	Discussion on benefits of participant-led antenatal classes	To educate parents about forthcoming labour, birth and beyond
	Discussion of mental health issues	To identify families at risk or in need of further support – if detected refer for additional support

Table 9.2: Advice to be given to women during the antenatal period

After looking at Table 9.2, you may need to refresh your own knowledge of fetal development, so you can share this with parents and show them the images and development of their growing fetus in *The Pregnancy Book* (DH, 2009) or other resources you may have. While the initial information sharing is important, women's experiences, emotions and circumstances can alter throughout pregnancy, so the initial assessment is not the only way a midwife determines which families need further support to promote positive parenting.

Ongoing antenatal care

Maternal and fetal wellbeing are assessed on 11 occasions (for a woman who has not had a baby before) and 9 occasions for previous mothers.

Activity 9.2   *Critical thinking*

With a friend see if you can recall the timing of the antenatal appointments offered to all pregnant women. Think about when you could promote parenting knowledge and advice during these meetings.

The answer regarding the routine antenatal visits can be found at the end of this chapter; the antenatal educational opportunities will be considered in the following paragraphs.

Now you have remembered the routine scheduling of antenatal care, we will consider how you can use these opportunities to enhance parenting knowledge. In addition to the table of advice and information offered above, NHS Health Scotland suggests parents are told the following information as this may promote fetal–parental interactions, which could have a benefit to the whole family (the link is at the end of this section). A midwife is best placed to offer this information during antenatal appointments to all parents.

- Babies are able to remember from the first trimester.
- Babies communicate through movement all the way through pregnancy.
- It is really important to communicate and stimulate a baby right from the start.
- Unborn babies can recognise their mum's voice from 16 weeks and their dad's from 20 weeks.
- Unborn babies respond to singing and being read to from 24 weeks. They may move about to show that they are listening.
- Babies develop preferences for music while in the uterus.
- They can move in rhythm to music and their heart rate increases.
- You can help to keep your baby happy and help it to develop in lots of ways before it is born:

  - stroke the tummy
  - sing
  - play music
  - expose your tummy to light, and
  - gentle vibrations.

- Talking to the unborn baby helps it to make sense of the world and start to link words and actions.
- Communicating with your unborn baby helps attachment and bonding.
- Mothers communicate non-verbally to their unborn babies through the way that they feel. Unborn babies are aware of how their mum feels, so try to control stress levels and take time to relax. Baby will love sharing this time with you!

This list has been reproduced from **www.maternal-and-early-years.org.uk/communication-in-the-antenatal-period**

Support in the antenatal period
Rights and benefits

The Child Health Promotion Programme (2008) explicitly states that preparation for parenthood begins with all (universal) prospective parents in early pregnancy and continues up to birth. This preparation includes maternal and paternal rights and benefits. In the UK the midwife usually completes the MatB1 form, a form which enables women to claim Statutory Maternity Pay from their employer or Maternity Allowance from the job centre if they are unemployed. The certificate verifies the pregnancy and expected date of delivery. The allowances are paid from 29 weeks' gestation for a maximum of 39 weeks. Conditions do apply, so if a woman is not eligible for these maternity allowances she may be able eligible for Employment and Support Allowance. In addition to these payments families on low incomes are eligible for a Sure Start Maternity Grant. Currently (January 2015) the payment for Maternity Allowance is: £138.18 a week or 90% of your average weekly earnings (whichever is lower). Statutory Maternity Pay is based on the woman's earnings but will be equivalent to or higher than Maternity Allowance. The Sure Start maternity grant is a one-off payment of £500.

While a woman is entitled to time off work for antenatal appointments, the fathers may have difficulty attending all the scheduled visits as there is no legal right for them to attend these visits. Some fathers may be able to negotiate time off and work later in the day to make up lost time. If we revisit the NICE (2008) antenatal care guidelines and The Child Health Promotion Programme (2008) we can see what is offered to all women and their partners.

Reviewing this table, you may need to see who is responsible for the antenatal review. In many areas this will be the health visiting team, and with the increase in health visitors nationally this may be happening for all women now. Over the last few years the number of families with

Who/when	What	Why
Before or at 36 weeks (NICE, 2008)	Offer breastfeeding information, including technique and good management practices that would help a woman succeed, such as detailed in the UNICEF 'Baby Friendly Initiative' (**www.babyfriendly.org.uk**)	To promote breastfeeding and support women to achieve this
	– preparation for labour and birth	For parents to be prepared for birth
	– care of the new baby	For information so parents can care for and make decisions after the birth of their baby
	– vitamin K prophylaxis	
	– newborn screening tests	
	– postnatal self-care	
	– awareness of 'baby blues' and postnatal depression.	

After 28 weeks (DH, 2008)	Promotion of ongoing health and wellbeing	Ongoing to identify families in need of additional support
	Parent's Guide to Money is distributed	To help families plan their finances
	Involvement of fathers	So fathers can support their partners, and care for their infants
	Antenatal review with Child Health Promotion Programme team	To focus on the emotional preparation for birth, carer–infant relationship, parenting and attachment
		Inform parents about infant development, distribute newborn screening information and sudden infant death syndrome guidance Distribute the Personal Child Health Record

Table 9.3: Ongoing support in pregnancy devised from NICE (2008) and CHPP (2009)

additional health and wellbeing needs who needed extra support were being seen by the health visitors but families with no additional needs did not always receive this review. Next time you are working in the community ask your mentor what happens in your local area.

Preparing for parenthood

While the antenatal visits/appointments are an opportunity to connect with the unborn baby, specific preparation for parenthood classes are designed to help mothers and fathers prepare for birth and beyond. NICE (2008) recommend all women and their partners are offered antenatal education at 34 weeks' gestation. Around the UK there are many antenatal programmes to prepare for and promote parenting on offer.

Activity 9.3   *Evidence-based practice*

With a colleague think about the antenatal education offered in your Trust. What does the programme entail; is there anything you feel is missing? Now look up the following website which offers suggested antenatal education: **www.nct.org.uk/sites/default/files/related_documents/1preparing-mothers-and-fathers-for-pregnancy-birth-and-beyond.pdf**

How does it differ from your local provision?

There are some possible answers at the end of the chapter.

The precise content of the classes may differ between areas and between facilitators but the principles include first and foremost social support. Meeting in groups can create informal networks between many couples. First time prospective parents often meet couples at a similar time in their pregnancy and this connection becomes an informal support network which continues long beyond the classes. Having one single session for parent education reduces the chance couples have to interact with others. Many people are initially shy of introducing themselves to others, but a facilitator can help with these introductions. Similarly, if classes are held over a number of weeks, the introductions may occur more spontaneously over the coffee breaks and in entrance halls as couples arrive. Next time you facilitate a class; see if you can help couples talk to others.

Relationship changes are considered during antenatal classes; inevitably a couple becoming a family or a family of three becoming four will have to make adjustments. Being aware of possible adjustments prior to the arrival of the new baby can help the transition to parenthood, or the expanding family. With the new arrival comes new responsibilities; a discussion about these may help couples minimise any tension that may occur as a result of these additional roles.

The parent–infant interaction is also an integral part of the antenatal education programme. During pregnancy healthcare professionals should focus time and attention to educating prospective parents about the important role interacting with their baby has.

If we refer back to the activity above and the National Childbirth Trust document you will see they state the benefits of antenatal education as being:

- Increased satisfaction with the experience of giving birth.
- Improved maternal health behaviours, such as reductions in smoking and alcohol consumption during pregnancy and increased uptake of breastfeeding.
- Greater confidence in parenting and understanding of relationships, both with their baby and between parents, particularly where programmes continue through pregnancy and into the early postnatal months.
- Well facilitated groups that support interactive learning are mixed and the right size can build valuable supportive social networks that continue after the life time of the group.

Antenatal education may be offered to groups of people with specific concerns, such as men only. These sessions can cover how men can support their partner during birth, care of the infant and emotional and practical fatherhood. In addition to these classes there are opportunities for young parenting programmes and classes delivered in languages other than English, to meet the needs of the local populations. Have a look and see what is available, possibly through your local Children's Centre next time you are in the community.

Breastfeeding

In addition to antenatal education, or perhaps as part of the education package, sessions on breastfeeding are promoted. The benefits of breastfeeding are extolled, but also practical help so women are aware of barriers to successful breastfeeding, including family members' lack of support. A UNICEF UK Baby Friendly Initiative and the Department of Health (2011) leaflet *Off to the Best Start* is a great introduction to the benefits of breastfeeding.

Activity 9.4   *Evidence-based practice*

Access the UNICEF and DH (2011) leaflet *Off to the Best Start:* **www.unicef.org.uk/ Documents/Baby_Friendly/Leaflets/otbs_leaflet.pdf**

Remind yourself of the benefits of breastfeeding in parent friendly language on pages 4 and 5. Do you know where this leaflet is at work, so you can use it when discussing feeding with prospective parents?

Then see if you can remind yourself of the best available evidence on breastfeeding bene-fits with this more in-depth link from UNICEF:

www.unicef.org.uk/BabyFriendly/News-and-Research/Research/Breastfeeding-research—An-overview/

Click on each topic for a range of supporting research.

This is an activity to familiarise yourself with up-to-date research; there is no specific question nor answers at the end of this chapter.

While you probably know many of the benefits of breastfeeding it is a good idea to check back to the UNICEF website frequently as new evidence is often posted and this will help keep you up to date.

www.unicef.org.uk/BabyFriendly/Resources/Guidance-for-Health-Professionals/ Forms-and-checklists/New-guidance-for-antenatal-and-postnatal-conversations

As a student midwife, you will be able to participate in antenatal education, but you will probably spend more time with women in labour and postnatally than at specific classes. You may be won-dering how this chapter fits into your role now.

Birth and beyond

The closer to term labour starts and a baby is born, the better the outcome for the baby and the transition to parenthood. A term baby usually has fewer problems adapting to extrauterine life; a preterm or low birth weight baby may need help in its transition. Let's think about the effects of a baby's birth on its future outcomes.

Activity 9.5   *Critical thinking*

With a colleague familiarise yourself with the following and their potential effect on neo-natal health and parenting: birth weight; birth trauma; birth asphyxia; preterm birth.

Potential answers are given at the end of the chapter.

Now you have considered the consequences of potential complications to birth, we will look at how a midwife can promote attachment and bonding in the majority of healthy term births.

After the birth

The introduction of a baby to extrauterine life, to being held and cared for by its parents has positive short- and long-term effects. Immediately after the birth of their baby, parents, often the mother, will be offered naked skin-to-skin contact. While skin-to-skin contact is a key factor in the establishment of breastfeeding it should be offered to all women regardless of their feeding intention as the benefits of this practice are numerous.

> ## Concept summary: Skin-to-skin contact
>
> - This contact helps keep the baby warm, a role the mother's uterus previously undertook.
> - It helps regulate the baby's heart rate and breathing, again activities the baby has to initiate once born, in their transition to extrauterine life.
> - The baby's blood sugar is more likely to be stable.
> - The baby is likely to cry less.
> - It enables the mother to touch and stroke her baby.

This positive introduction then leads to the mother showing and feeling greater confidence in caring for her quiet, warm baby and initiating breastfeeding. The midwife, or student, can help this initial bonding between the mother, or father, and their baby by saying how content the baby is, by commenting on its quiet nature and by reinforcing the positive benefits of this early skin-to-skin contact. This contact is not a one-time activity but can be used at home over the next few months and beyond to calm a baby and to enhance the attachment between the baby and parents.

Practices that support this transition to parenting include a quiet birthing environment, with dim lighting; drug and intervention free labour and births, where possible; minimal separation of the baby from its mother and a supportive midwife. The midwife can also help once the baby starts to demonstrate pre-feeding cues. These are movements the baby makes towards breastfeeding. A mother who chooses to bottle feed her baby should be educated about these cues too, so she can initiate the feeding method of her choice. This leaflet contains all the essential information about bottle feeding a newborn baby: **www.unicef.org.uk/BabyFriendly/Parents/Resources/Resources-for-parents/A-guide-to-infant-formula-for-parents-who-are-bottle-feeding**

Neonatal feeding cues are quite subtle and may include the following: sucking movements and noises, lip licking, head movements from side to side, rapid eye movements and restlessness. Crying is considered to be a late sign of hunger and not the first sign a baby needs feeding. Recognising early feeding cues and offering the breast or bottle, if preferred, may help initiate feeding. Teaching a new mother about these cues will enable her to respond to them before the baby starts to cry. Feeding on demand, unrestricted or baby led feeding; responding to their cues is considered good practice. On average babies feed about eight times in 24 hours. Feeding as and when the baby is ready is beneficial as it ensures an adequate milk supply is available, there is less infant weight loss in the first few days, increased duration of breastfeeding and prevents common problems which undermine women's confidence in their feeding ability. As a midwife you should ensure all parents have the best available information on feeding their baby.

A quick reminder of advice you can use to reassure parents that their baby is getting sufficient milk:

- They appear content and satisfied after most feeds.
- They are healthy and gaining weight after the first two weeks.
- Your breasts and nipples should not be sore.
- After the first few days, your baby should have at least six wet nappies a day.
- After the first few days they should also pass at least two yellow stools every day.

For more specific information access this document:

www.unicef.org.uk/Documents/Baby_Friendly/Going%20Baby%20Friendly/Mothers_ breastfeeding_checklist.pdf?epslanguage=en

When parents are reassured their baby is feeding well their confidence in their parenting ability is reinforced. While the biological aspects of breastfeeding for the mother and baby are well publicised, the role of breastfeeding in building a relationship between the mother and child is less so.

This relational aspect of breastfeeding includes the physical closeness breastfeeding affords, enabling frequent skin-to-skin contact several times a day in addition to the benefits of the hormones produced. Oxytocin is associated with sensitive care giving (Rilling, 2013). Oxytocin and prolactin respectively are called hormones of love and calm; these are desirable in parenting, especially in the early transition period which is sometimes one of uncertainty.

The distance from the baby's face when at the breast to the mother's face is optimal for their sight. Facial expressions and eye contact shared between the mother and baby are the first stages in the baby's communication development (Sullivan *et al.*, 2011). Having this understanding can also help fathers to replicate this distance so they too can smile, talk and look at their baby to promote this interaction and bond with them. Babies hear voices and will vocalise themselves in their innate need to make a connection to others for their care.

Parents can be supported in bonding with their baby with this knowledge and bonding can be enhanced by activities such as wearing a baby in a sling and increasing the amount of times they touch their baby (Sullivan *et al.*, 2011), either through skin-to-skin contact or infant massage. Wearing a baby in a sling helps infants develop emotionally, as they are close to their care giver, and socially as they see the world around them. Babies are often quieter as they are soothed by the motion and closeness of others, which mimics their experience in utero, hearing the mother's heart beat and voice. Babies can sleep in the sling during the day while the parents can continue with their other responsibilities, whether this is preparing a meal or caring for other children. Many Children's Centres offer infant massage classes, where parents can learn these skills and meet other new parents too. The benefits of infant massage include: improving the baby's circulation, sensory awareness, relaxation, neurological development, and bonding between parents and child.

Another controversial approach to promoting infant–parent bonding is co-sleeping or bed sharing. While the evidence for improving breastfeeding duration while co-sleeping is not in doubt, the practice is a risk for sudden infant death syndrome (SIDS). As midwifery students you are used to recommending that babies sleep in their own cot, next to the parent's bed. The baby should be on their back with their feet at the foot of the cot. To maximise parental decision-making about where the baby sleeps, and to prevent SIDS, UNICEF has produced the following statement for health professionals.

UNICEF statement on bed sharing

Simplistic messages in relation to where a baby sleeps should be avoided; neither blanket prohibitions nor blanket permissions reflect the current research evidence.

The current body of evidence overwhelmingly supports the following key messages, which should be conveyed to all parents:

- The safest place for your baby to sleep is in a cot by your bed.
- Sleeping with your baby on a sofa puts your baby at greatest risk.
- Your baby should not share a bed with anyone who:
  - is a smoker;
  - has consumed alcohol;
  - has taken drugs (legal or illegal) that make them sleepy.

The incidence of SIDS (often called 'cot death') is higher in the following groups:

- Parents in low socioeconomic groups.
- Parents who currently abuse alcohol or drugs.
- Young mothers with more than one child.
- Premature infants and those with low birth weight.

Parents within these groups will need more face-to-face discussion to ensure that these key messages are explored and understood. They may need some practical help, possibly from other agencies, to enable them to put them into practice.

www.unicef.org.uk/BabyFriendly/News-and-Research/News/UNICEF-UK-Baby-Friendly-Initiative-statement-on-new-bed-sharing-research

You may notice from the statement above that most of the chapters covered in this book are concerned with women or parents who fall into the higher risk groups. It is therefore your responsibility to ensure they understand the safest place for their baby to sleep. This UNICEF document helps parents understand the best available evidence for caring for their baby at night: **www.unicef.org.uk/Documents/Baby_Friendly/Leaflets/caringatnight_web.pdf**

Caring for a baby during the day is sometimes easier than during the night when parents are tired and their decision-making capabilities or their empathy to their baby may be impaired. Discussing parental concerns at every postnatal visit is essential for determining the parents' coping and caring mechanisms. In addition to asking about baby feeding, sleeping and waking times the midwife will review the baby to determine it is healthy as per NICE (2014b) postnatal guidelines. This includes looking for signs of jaundice, which may need treatment, and supporting parents and offering resolution if their baby is constipated, has nappy rash, has colic or is unwell.

Ongoing breastfeeding or bottle feeding support is offered at every contact. This ensures the parents are supported and informed of the best available evidence to feed their baby safely. A midwifery support worker may also be asked to support parents with infant feeding concerns whether these stem from breastfeeding issues or ability to make a safe formula feed.

The NICE (2014b) postnatal guidance says midwives should assess emotional attachment and promote parent–baby interactions. There is a need to support both the mother and the father so they can both understand the importance of their eye contact, socialisation with and responses to their baby to optimise their development. Parents too should be encouraged to join social networks for their own support and social interactions. Group based parenting programmes should be offered to parents when midwives are concerned about the parents' ability to respond compassionately to their baby.

Around 10 days postnatally, the health visiting team take over the care of the family from the midwife; they continue to promote positive family interactions and are alert for signs of stress or need in families. The terms universal and progressive are used to identify practice that is offered to all families and other support offered to those considered in need of a higher level of support.

The absence of sensitive care from a consistent caregiver in very early life can result in severely disordered emotional and social development. Lack of positive attention and supervision by parents, and inconsistent, harsh or inappropriate discipline are causes of antisocial behaviour, conduct disorder (the most common childhood disability), criminality, delinquency and violence.

Child abuse (emotional, sexual and physical) and neglect impacts on mental health, and can cause depression, post-traumatic stress disorder, personality disorder and low self-esteem in later life. It is responsible for an average of two child deaths each week in the UK.

While this chapter is concerned with promoting parenting, in the absence of a strong attachment to the child and emotional resources of the parent, child abuse is a potential threat to babies. This can be non-accidental, emotional or physical neglect or sexual in nature. Undertake Activity 9.6 to see the prevalence of death from abuse or neglect with babies under 1 year of age.

Activity 9.6   *Evidence-based practice*

Look on the National Society for the Prevention of Cruelty to Children (NSPCC) website. You will find a report on serious case reviews for children under 1 year of age. A serious case review is a review of the professional input in cases where children die.

www.nspcc.org.uk/Inform/resourcesforprofessionals/underones/under_ones_ scr_analysis_wda86352.html

There are no answers at the end of this chapter as the information which follows is related to this activity.

The analysis of the 130 infants, who died in England and Wales since 2008, included 60 cases where domestic abuse was a factor, 46 where substance misuse was a factor and 34 where parental mental health was a factor. Therefore, supporting the inclusion of these groups of prospective parents into an intensive parenting programme is recommended. While these are the infants who died, there are estimates for the number of babies living in vulnerable and complex family situations.

Concept summary: Babies at risk

According to the same NSPCC document, in the UK an estimated:

- 19,500 babies under 1-year-old are living with a parent who has used Class A drugs in the last year.
- 39,000 babies under 1-year-old live in households affected by domestic violence in the last year.
- 93,500 babies under 1-year-old live with a parent who is a problem drinker.
- 144,000 babies under 1-year-old live with a parent who has a common mental health problem.

The Child Health Promotion Programme (CHPP; DH, 2008) has initiatives for parents with the problems identified in the above concept summary under their progressive programme. Promoting sensitive parenting is a priority for all parents, using resources such as *The Social Baby* book (Murray and Andrews, 2005).

If the parents have one of the above identified difficulties or other associated needs the following table taken from the CHPP states the care the parents should be offered.

If you or the health visiting team notice any insensitive, intrusive or passive parenting interactions, referral to other services as soon as possible promotes the best opportunity for the baby's emotional, social and psychological milestone development.

Higher risk	Offer
At risk first time young mothers	Individualised evidence based programmes such as the Family Nurse Partnership Multimodal support combining home visiting, like skills training and integration within social networks
Parents with learning difficulties	Information on support available to the parents Multi-agency support should include individual, group based and home visiting Further specific support might include speech and language therapy
Drug and alcohol misuse	Refer one or both parents to local specialist services CHPP team to contribute to care package led by specialists
Domestic abuse	Follow local guidelines Provision of a safe environment so victims can discuss concerns Sources of support for victims
Serious mental illness	Refer one or both parents to specialist mental health services CHPP team to contribute to care package led by specialists
Parents in conflict	Refer to parenting groups which address conflict resolution training
Women whose first language is not English	Refer to English as a second language services

Table 9.4: What care should parents with particular needs be offered?
Source: CHPP.

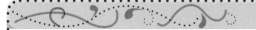

Chapter summary

This chapter has focused on activities and information midwives can suggest to enhance the infant–parent interactions before and after birth. The development of the fetus is influenced by many factors during pregnancy from stress to chemical harm caused by smoking, alcohol or drug misuse and bacteria which can be avoided such as listeriosis. During pregnancy fetal growth is measured as an indicator of fetal development and wellbeing as well as maternal observations. The aim of these activities is to identify women and fetuses at risk. Antenatal education helps prepare parents for birth and the change to their family dynamics. Couples who are prepared for this transition may cope better with the early days of parenthood.

A healthy neonate has the optimum chance at normal development; risks such as prematurity or birth trauma may be transient or long term. Promoting positive interactions between all women and their babies can be offered in early skin-to-skin contact. This increased the success of breastfeeding which has many benefits both physical and relational. In the postnatal period a midwife assesses other concerns and refers families or their babies for additional care or support, depending on their unique circumstances. The role of the midwife includes noticing and supporting or referring poor parenting interactions, safeguarding neonates, offering information on safe sleeping practices and handing over care to the health visitor and other agencies. The families covered in the rest of this book may benefit from extra support in their transition to parenthood.

Activities: brief outline answers

Activity 9.2 Critical thinking [page 167]

For a woman who is nulliparous with an uncomplicated pregnancy, a schedule of ten appointments should be adequate. For a woman who is parous with an uncomplicated pregnancy, a schedule of seven appointments should be adequate.

Nulliparous women are offered their first appointment ideally by 10 weeks. Then further appointments at 16 weeks, 25 weeks, 28, 31, 34, 36, 38, 40 and 41 weeks.

Multiparous women are offered the same except not the 25, 31 or 40 week appointments.

All women are also offered an ultrasound between 18–20 weeks' gestation.

Activity 9.3 Evidence-based practice [page 169]

The NCT suggests six sessions focusing on the development of the unborn baby, changes for me and us, our/my health and wellbeing, giving birth and meeting our baby, caring for my/our new baby and who is there for us, services and people.

Your Trust may not offer six classes, but a one day intensive programme. It may concentrate more on the birth than the pregnancy and services after birth.

Activity 9.5 Critical thinking [page 171]

Birth weight: this is divided into two groups of babies.

Large or macrosomic babies who weigh over 4.5 kg and may be due to maternal diabetes. These babies are at risk of hypoglycaemia following birth and may have had a greater risk of birth trauma due to their size.

Small for gestational age babies are those whose weight plotted on a centile chart is below the 10th centile for their gestation – they can be term or preterm. These babies are at risk of hypothermia, hypoglycaemia and jaundice; more care, observations and sometimes interventions are required.

Birth trauma: results from difficult births, perhaps shoulder dystocia, breech, operative birth or emergency caesarean section for fetal reasons. The initial attachment with the parents can be disrupted by medical interventions.

Birth asphyxia: monitoring of the fetus in utero and the neonate following birth can determine whether a baby has been deprived of oxygen. Signs of asphyxia include pathological CTG trace accompanied by fetal blood sampling and/or low Apgar score (below 3) and poor cord gases.

Preterm birth: the shorter the pregnancy duration the greater the incidence of neonatal problems requiring medical and nursing interventions. Respiratory distress, bronchopulmonary dysplasia, hypoglycaemia, hypothermia, jaundice, neonatal infections and developmental delay are complications.

Further reading

DH (2008) *The Child Health Promotion Programme*. London: Crown Copyright. (Available to download at **www.rcn.org.uk/__data/assets/pdf_file/0009/155889/286448_ChildHealth_acc.pdf**)

DH (2009) *The Pregnancy Book*. London: Department of Health.

Faculty of Public Health (2005) *Parenting and Public Health Briefing Statement.* London: Faculty of Public Health.

Useful paper to remind professionals of existing knowledge. (Available to download at **www.fph. org.uk/uploads/bs_parenting.pdf**).

Murray, L. and Andrews, L. (2005) *The Social Baby.* London: CP Publishing.

Useful websites

The National Childbirth Trust **www.nct.org.uk**

UK-based charity supporting new parents and parents-to-be.

UNICEF UK Baby Friendly Initiative **www.unicef.org.uk/babyfriendly**

Useful source of leaflets and parent-friendly information.

References

Advisory Council on the Misuse of Drugs [ACMD] (2011) *Hidden Harm: Responding to the Needs of Children of Problem Drug Users*. www.gov.uk/government/uploads/system/uploads/attachment_data/file/120620/hidden-harm-full.pdf, accessed 20 February 2015.

Ameh, C.A. and van den Broek, N. (2008) Increased risk of maternal death among ethnic minority women in the UK. *Obstetrician and Gynaecologist*, 10(3): 177–182.

Annon, J. (1976) The PLISSIT model: a proposed conceptual scheme for the behavioural treatment of sexual problems. *Journal of Sex Education Therapy*, 2(1): 1–15.

Anorexia and Bulimia Care. www.anorexiabulimiacare.org.uk, accessed 20 February 2015.

Antonovsky, A. (1979) *Health, Stress and Coping*. San Francisco: Jossey-Bass.

APA (2013) *Diagnostic and Statistical Manual of Mental Health Disorders* 5. Arlington, VA: American Psychiatric Association.

Arroll, B., Goodyear-Smith, F., Kerse, N., *et al.* (2005). Effect of the addition of a 'help' question to two screening questions on specificity for diagnosis of depression in general practice: diagnostic validity study. *British Medical Journal* 331: 884.

Ashmead, G.G. (2003) Smoking and pregnancy. *Journal of Maternal-Fetal and Neonatal Medicine*, 14(5): 297–304.

Aveyard, P., Lawrence, T., Croghan, E., Evans, O. and Cheng, K.K. (2005) Is advice to stop smoking from a midwife stressful for pregnant women who smoke? Data from a randomised controlled trial. *Preventative Medicine*, 40(5): 572–582.

Babor, T.F., Higgins-Biddle, J.C., Saunders, J.B. and Monteiro, M.G. (2001) A*UDIT: the Alcohol Use Disorders Identification Test: Guidelines for Use in Primary Care*, 2nd edn. WHO/MSD/MSB/01.6a Switzerland, World Health Organisation, www.talkingalcohol.com/files/pdfs/WHO_audit.pdf, accessed 20 February 2015.

Bacchus, L., Bewley, S. and Mezey, G. (2001) Domestic violence in pregnancy. *Fetal and Maternal Medicine Review*, 12: 249–271.

Baggaley, R. (2008) *HIV for Non-HIV Specialists: Diagnosing the Undiagnosed*. London: Medical Foundation for AIDS and Sexual Health.

Barrett, G., Pendry, E., Peacock, J., Victor, C.R. and Thackar, R. (2000) Women's sexual health after childbirth. *British Journal of Obstetrics and Gynaecology*, 107: 186–195.

BASHH (2014a) *United Kingdom National Guideline on the Management of Trichomonas vaginalis*, www.bashh.org/documents/UK%20national%20guideline%20on%20the%20management%20of%20TV%20%202014.pdf, accessed 20 February 2015.

BASHH (2014b) *British Association for Sexual Health and HIV: Clinical Guidance*, www.bashh.org/BASHH/Guidelines/Guidelines/BASHH/Guidelines/Guidelines.aspx, accessed 20 February 2015.

Bateman, B. and Simpson, L. (2006) Higher rate of stillbirth at the extremes of reproductive age: a large nationwide sample of deliveries in the United States. *American Journal of Obstetrics and Gynecology*, 194(3): 840–845.

BBC Newsbeat (2014) Young mothers face stigma and abuse, say charities. www.bbc.co.uk/newsbeat/26326035, accessed 20 February 2015.

B-eat (2012) *Costs of Eating Disorders in England: Economic Impacts of Anorexia Nervosa, Bulimia Nervosa and Other Disorders, Focussing on Young People.* https://www.b-eat.co.uk/assets/000/000/146/CostsofEating DisordersinEnglandReport_original.pdf?1403538000, accessed 20 February 2015.

Beauchamp, T. and Childress, J. (2012) *Principles of Biomedical Ethics,* 7th edn. Oxford: Oxford University Press.

Beecher Bryant, H. (2011) *The Experience of Midwives Report.* London: Maternity Action.

BHIVA (2014) British HIV Association guidelines for the management of HIV infection in pregnant women 2012 (2014 interim review). *HIV Medicine* 15 (Suppl. 4): 1–77. www.bhiva.org/documents/ Guidelines/Pregnancy/2012/BHIVA-Pregnancy-guidelines-update-2014.pdf, accessed 20 February 2015.

Biro, M.A., Davey, M., Carolan, M. and Kealy, M. (2012) Advanced maternal age and obstetric morbidity for women giving birth in Victoria, Australia: a population-based study. *Australian and New Zealand Journal of Obstetrics and Gynaecology,* 52(3): 229–234.

BMA (2004) *Smoking and Reproductive Health: The Impact of Smoking on Sexual, Reproductive and Child Health.* London: BMA.

Bollini, P., Pampallona, S., Wanner, P. and Kupelnick, B. (2009) Pregnancy outcome of migrant women and integration policy: a systematic review of the international literature. *Social Science and Medicine,* 68(3): 452–461.

Bornstein, M.H., Putnick, D.L., Suwalsky, T.D. and Gini, M. (2006) Maternal chronological age, prenatal and perinatal history, social support and parenting of infants. *Child Development,* 77(4): 875–892.

Brealey, S., Hewitt, C., Green, J.M., *et al.* (2010) Screening for postnatal depression – is it acceptable to women and healthcare professionals? A systematic review and meta-synthesis. *Journal of Reproductive and Infant Psychology,* 28(4): 328–344.

British Medical Association (1998) *Domestic Violence: A Health Care Issue?* London: BMA.

British Obesity Surgery Patient Association (2014) www.bospauk.org, accessed 20 February 2015.

Broecke, S. and Hamed, J. (2008) *Gender Gaps in Higher Education Participation.* London: Department of Innovation, Universities and Skills Research Report 08 14.

Butland, B., Jebb, S., Kopelman, P., McPherson, K., Thomas, S., Mardell, J. and Parry, V. (2007) *Foresight. Tackling Obesities: Future Choices.* Project report. London: Government Office for Science.

Byrne, L., Townsend, C.L., Thorne, C. and Tookey, P.A. (2013) *Place of Diagnosis and CD4 Count in Pregnant HIV-Positive Women Diagnosed Before Conception in the UK and Ireland (2007–2012) (Poster).* 19th Annual Conference of the British HIV Association (BHIVA 2013), Manchester, UK.

Byrom, A. (2004) Advanced maternal age: a literature review. *British Journal of Midwifery,* 12(12): 779–783.

Carolan, M. (2010) Pregnancy health status of sub-Saharan refugee women who have resettled in developed countries: a review of the literature. *Midwifery,* 26(4): 407–414.

Carolan, M. (2013) Maternal age ≥45 years and maternal and perinatal outcomes: a review of the evidence. *Midwifery,* 29(5): 479–489.

Carson, C., Redshaw, M., Quigley, M.A., *et al.* (2013) Effects of pregnancy planning, fertility, and assisted reproductive treatment on child behavioral problems at 5 and 7 years: evidence from the Millennium Cohort Study. *Fertility and Sterility,* 99(2): 456–463.

Centre for Maternal and Child Enquiries (CMACE) (2011) Saving mothers' lives: reviewing maternal deaths to make motherhood safer: 2006–08. The Eighth Report on Confidential Enquiries into Maternal Deaths in the United Kingdom. *BJOG* 118(Suppl. 1): 1–203.

References

Chamberlain, C., O'Mara-Eves, A., Oliver, S., Caird, J.R., Perlen, S.M., Eades, S.J. and Thomas, J. (2013) Psychosocial interventions for supporting women to stop smoking in pregnancy. *Cochrane Database of Systematic Reviews*, 2013, Issue 10. Art. No. CD001055. DOI: 10.1002/14651858.CD001055.pub4; http://summaries.cochrane.org/CD001055/PREG_psychosocial-interventions-for-supporting-women-to-stop-smoking-in-pregnancy, accessed 20 February 2015.

Claesson, I.-M., Klein, S., Gunilla Sydsjö, G., *et al.* (2014) Physical activity and psychological well-being in obese pregnant and postpartum women attending a weight-gain restriction programme. *Midwifery*, 30(1): 11–16.

Cleary-Goldman, J., Malone, F.D., Vidaver, J., *et al.* (2005) Impact of maternal age on obstetric outcome. *Obstetrics and Gynecology*, 105(5 Part 1): 983–990.

Coad, J. and Dunstall, M. (2012) *Anatomy and Physiology for Midwives*, 3rd edn. Edinburgh: Churchill Livingstone.

Coe, C. and Barlow, J. (2013) Supporting women with perinatal mental health problems: the role of the voluntary sector. *Community Practitioner*, 86(2): 23–27.

Coid, J., Yang, M., Roberts, A., *et al.* (2006) Violence and psychiatric morbidity in the national household population of Britain: public health implications. *British Journal of Psychiatry*. DOI: 10.1192/bjp.189.1.12.

Conde-Agudelo, A., Rosas-Bermudez, A. and Kafury-Goeta, A.C. (2006) Birth spacing and risk of adverse perinatal outcomes: a meta-analysis. *JAMA*, 295: 1809–1823.

Cooke, A., Mills, T.A. and Lavender, T. (2011) Advanced maternal age: delayed childbearing is rarely a conscious choice. *International Journal of Nursing Studies*, 49: 30–39.

Correa, S. (2014) Is caseload midwifery care the best practice? A review of the literature. *MIDIRS Midwifery Digest*, 24(4): 431–435.

Council of Europe (2002) *Recommendation Rec (2002)5 of the Committee of Ministers to Member States on the Protection against Violence Adopted on 30 April 2002 and Explanatory Memorandum.* Strasbourg: Council of Europe.

Delbaere, I., Verstraelen, H., Goetgeluk, S., Martens, G., De Backer, G. and Temmerman, M. (2007) Pregnancy outcome in primiparae of advanced maternal age. *European Journal of Obstetrics and Gynecology and Reproductive Biology*, 135(1): 41–46.

Department for Children, Schools and Families [DCSF] (2007) *Teenage Parents Next Steps: Guidance for Local Authorities and Primary Care Trusts*, www.changeforchildren.co.uk/uploads/Teenage_Pregnancy_Next_Steps_For_LAs_And_PCTs.pdf, accessed 20 February 2015.

Department for Children, Schools and Families [DCSF] (2008) *Teenage Parents: Who Cares? A Guide to Commissioning and Delivering Maternity Services for Young Parents*, 2nd edn; http://webarchive.nationalarchives.gov.uk/20130401151715/https://www.education.gov.uk/publications/standard/Childrenandfamilies/Page11/DCSF-00414-2008, accessed 20 February 2015.

Department for Children, Schools and Families [DCSF] (2010) *Teenage Pregnancy Strategy: Beyond 2010.* www.education.gov.uk/consultations/downloadableDocs/4287_Teenage%20pregnancy%20strategy_aw8.pdf, accessed 20 February 2015.

Department of Health [DH] (2001) *The National Strategy for Sexual Health and HIV.* London: Department of Health.

Department of Health [DH/DFeS] (2004) *National Service Framework for Children, Young People and Maternity Services.* London: Department of Health/Department for Education and Skills.

Department of Health [DH] (2007) *Review of the Health Inequalities Infant Mortality PSA Target.* London: Department of Health.

Department of Health [DH] (2008) *The Child Health Promotion Programme: Pregnancy and the First Five Years of Life.* London: Department of Health/Department for Children, Schools and Families.

Department of Health [DH] (2009) *The Pregnancy Book.* London: Department of Health.

Department of Health [DH] (2010) *Midwifery 2020: Delivering Expectations.* London: Department of Health.

Department of Health [DH] (2012) *Compassion in Practice Nursing, Midwifery and Care Staff: Our Vision and Strategy.* London: HMSO.

Department of Health [DH] (2013a) *NHS Constitution and Values.* London: HMSO.

Department of Health [DH] (2013b) *A Framework for Sexual Health Improvement in England (Best Practice Guidance).* London: Department of Health.

Department of Health [DH] (2013c) *Helping People Make Informed Choices about Health and Social Care.* London: Department of Health.

Directive 2005/36/EC (2005) Article 42 of the European Parliament and of the Council of 7 September 2005 on the recognition of professional qualifications. *Official Journal of the European Union*, 255: 22–142.

Draycott, T., Lewis, G., Stephens, I., *et al.* (2011) Executive Summary; Centre for Maternal and Child Enquiries (CMACE). *BJOG*, 118(Suppl.1): e12–e21.

Dunn, C., Darnell, D., Carmel, A., *et al.* (2014) Comparing the motivational interviewing integrity in two prevalent models of brief intervention service delivery for primary care settings. *Journal of Substance Abuse Treatment*, DOI: 10.10.6/jsat2014.10.009 [Epub ahead of print].

Easter, A., Bye, A., Taborelli, E., Corfield, F., Schmidt, U., Treasure, J. and Micali, N. (2013) Recognising the symptoms: how common are eating disorders in pregnancy? *European Eating Disorders Review*, 21: 340–344. DOI: 10.1002/erv.2229.

Eastham, R. and Gosakan, R. (2010) Review smoking and smoking cessation in pregnancy. *The Obstetrician and Gynaecologist*, 12(21): 103–109.

Ecker, J. (2014) Harvard School of Public Health, http://theforum.sph.harvard.edu/events/delaying-pregnancy-and-parenthood, accessed 21 February 2015.

Edge, V. and Laros, R. (1993) Pregnancy outcome in nulliparous women aged 35 or older. *American Journal of Obstetrics and Gynecology*, 168(1): 1881–1885.

Everett-Murphy, K., Paijmans, J., Steyn, K., *et al.* (2011). Scolders, carers or friends: South African midwives' contrasting styles of communication when discussing smoking cessation with pregnant women. *Midwifery*, 27(4): 517–524.

Ewles, L. and Simnett, I. (2010) *Promoting Health: A Practical Guide.* London: Balliere Tindall Elsevier.

Faculty of Sexual and Reproductive Healthcare Clinical Effectiveness Unit (2009) *Postnatal Sexual and Reproductive Health*, www.fsrh.org/pdfs/CEUGuidancePostnatal09.pdf, accessed 21 February 2015.

Faculty of Sexual and Reproductive Healthcare Clinical Effectiveness Unit (2011) *Emergency Contraception.* www.fsrh.org/pdfs/CEUguidanceEmergencyContraception11.pdf, accessed 21 February 2015.

Faculty of Sexual and Reproductive Healthcare Clinical Effectiveness Unit (2013) *Use of Ulipristal Acetate (ellaOne®) in Breastfeeding Women.* Update from the Clinical Effectiveness Unit; www.fsrh.org/pdfs/CEUstatementUPAandBreastfeeding.pdf, accessed 21 February 2015.

References

Family Nurse Partnership (2015) *Research and Development,* http://fnp.nhs.uk/research-and-development, accessed 21 February 2015.

Family Planning Association (no date) *Contraceptive Help,* www.fpa.org.uk/help-and-advice/contraception-help; *My Contraceptive Tool,* www.fpa.org.uk/contraception-help/my-contraception-tool, accessed 21 February 2015.

Fish, J. (2009) *Cervical Screening in Lesbian and Bisexual Women: A Review of the Worldwide Literature Using Systematic Methods: De Montford University,* www.cancerscreening.nhs.uk/cervical/publications/screening-lesbians-bisexual-women.pdf, accessed 21 February 2015.

Forrester, M.B. and Merz, R.D. (2003) Maternal age-specific Down syndrome rates by maternal race/ethnicity, Hawaii: 1986–2000. *Birth Defects Research,* 67(9): 625–629.

Free Dictionary (2015) Definition of empowerment. Available at: www.thefreedictionary.com/empowerment, accessed 21 February 2015.

Gilbert, W., Nesbitt, T. and Danielsen, B. (1999) Childbearing beyond age 40: pregnancy outcome in 24,032 cases. *Obstetrics and Gynecology,* 93(1): 9–14.

Gingerbread (2014) *What Not to Say to a Single Parent,* http://gingerbread.org.uk/content/2051/What-not-to-say-to-a-single-parent, accessed 21 February 2015.

Glasier, A., McNeilly, A.S. and Howie, P.W. (1988) Hormonal background of lactational infertility. *International Journal of Fertility,* 33(Suppl): 32–34.

Glasier, A.F., Logan, J. and McGrew, T.J. (1996) Who gives advice about postpartum contraception? *Contraception,* 53: 217–220.

Goverde, H.J., Dekker, H.S., Janssen, H.J., Bastiaans, B.A., Rolland, R. and Zielhuis, G.A. (1995) Semen quality and frequency of smoking and alcohol consumption – an explorative study. *International Journal of Fertility and Menopausal Studies,* 40(3): 135–138. http://europepmc.org/abstract/MED/7663540, accessed 21 February 2015.

Green, J. and Tones, K. (2010) *Health Promotion: Planning and Strategies.* London: SAGE.

Greenhouse, P. (1995) A definition of sexual health. *BMJ,* 310: 1468.

Guillebaud, J. and MacGregor, A. (2013) *Contraception: Your Questions Answered,* 6th edn. Edinburgh: Elsevier.

Gupta, N., Kiran, U. and Bhal, K. (2008) Teenage pregnancies: obstetric characteristics and outcome. *European Journal of Obstetrics, Gynaecology and Reproductive Biology,* 137(2): 165–171.

Haith-Cooper, M. and Bradshaw, G. (2013) Meeting the health and social needs of pregnant asylum seekers, midwifery students' perspectives: Part 1: dominant discourses and midwifery students. *Nurse Education Today,* 33(9): 1008–1013.

Hall, A. (2012) Health promotion: to educate or empower? *British Journal of Midwifery,* 20(3): 156–156.

Harris, A. A. and Barger, M.K. (2010) Specialized care for women pregnant after bariatric surgery. *Journal of Midwifery and Women's Health,* 55(6): 529–539.

Harvey, S.T., Fisher, L.J., Kudzmaet, E.C., *et al.* (2012) Evaluating the clinical efficacy of a primary care-focused, nurse-led, consultation liaison model for perinatal mental health. *International Journal of Mental Health Nursing,* 21(1): 75–81.

Hatem, M., Sandall, J., Devane, D., *et al.* (2008) Midwife-led versus other models of care for childbearing women. *Cochrane Database of Systematic Reviews,* 4.

Haughney, P. (2012) *SMART Goals,* www.projectsmart.co.uk/smart-goals.html, accessed 21 February 2015.

Hawkes, S. and Gomez, G. (2013) Screening for syphilis in pregnancy: UK National Screening Committee, www.screening.nhs.uk/policydb_download.php?doc=359, accessed 21 February 2015.

Health and Social Care Information Centre [HSCIC] (2010) Infant Feeding Survey, November 2012, www.hscic.gov.uk, accessed 21 February 2015.

Health and Social Care Information Centre [HSCIC] (2014a) *Statistics on Women's Smoking Status at Time of Delivery, England. Quarter 1 2014–2015*, www.hscic.gov.uk, accessed 21 February 2015.

Health and Social Care Information Centre [HSCIC] (2014b) *Eating Disorders: Hospital Admissions Up by 8 Per Cent in a Year*, www.hscic.gov.uk, accessed 20 February 2015.

Henderson, J., Gao, H., Redshaw, M., *et al.* (2013) Experiencing maternity care: the care received and perceptions of women from different ethnic groups. *BMC Pregnancy Childbirth*, 22(13): 196.

Hicks, T.L., Goodall, S.F., Quattrone, E.M. and Lydon-Rocelle, M.T. (2004) Postpartum sexual functioning and method of delivery: summary of the evidence. *Journal of Midwifery and Women's Health*, 49(5): 430–436.

HIV-positive women in UK and Irish hospitals, 2008–2013. BHIVA Conference Presentation. *HIV Medicine*, 15(3): 2.

Hoffman, M.C., Jeffers, S., Carter, J., Duthely, L., Cotter, A. and Gonzalez-Quintero, V.H. (2007) Pregnancy at or beyond age 40 years is associated with an increased risk of fetal death and other adverse outcomes. *American Journal of Obstetrics and Gynecology*, 196(5): e11–e13.

Hoggart, L. and Phillips, J. (2010) *Young People in London: Abortion and Repeat Abortion*. London: Government Office for London.

Hollier, L., Leveno, K., Kelly, M., Mcintire, D. and Cunningham, F. (2000) Maternal age and malformations in singleton births. *Obstetrics and Gynecology*, 96(5 Part 1): 701–706.

Home Office (2013) *Domestic Violence and Abuse*, www.gov.uk/domestic-violence-and-abuse, accessed 21 February 2015.

Hood, S. (2014) How can midwives enhance experiences of maternity care for nulliparous women of advanced maternal age? Unpublished dissertation submitted as part of BSc(Hons) Midwifery, Ipswich, University Campus Suffolk.

Howard, L.M., Oram, S., Galley, H., *et al.* (2013) Domestic violence and perinatal mental disorders: a systematic review and meta-analysis. *Plos Medicine*, 10(5): e1001452–e1001452.

Humphreys, C. and Thiara, R. (2002) *Routes to Safety: Protection Issues Facing Abused Women and Children and the Role of Outreach Services*. Bristol: Women's Aid Federation of England.

Hunt, S. and Symonds, A. (1995) *The Social Meaning of Midwifery*. Hampshire: Macmillan.

Hunt, S.C. and Martin, A. (2001) *Pregnant Women: Violent Men: What Midwives Need to Know*. Oxford: Books for Midwives.

Hunter, L. (2013) Discourses of teenage motherhood: finding a framework that enables provision of appropriate support. Part 1: Risk discourses and the shortcomings of the Teenage Pregnancy Strategy and Part 2: Situational and developmental perspectives. *Essentially MIDIRS*, 4(4): 32–37.

Jacobi, C., Hayward, C., DeZwaan, M., Kraemer, H.C. and Agras, W.S. (2004) Coming to terms with risk factors for eating disorders: application of risk terminology and suggestions for a general taxonomy. *Psychological Bulletin*, 130: 19–65.

Jarrett, P. (2014) Attitudes of student midwives caring for women with perinatal mental health problems. *British Journal of Midwifery*, 22(10): 718–724.

Jayaweera, H. and Quigley, M.A. (2010) Health status, health behaviour and healthcare use among migrants in the UK: evidence from mothers in the Millennium Cohort Study. *Social Science and Medicine*, 71(5): 1002–1010.

Jefferies, J. (2008) Fertility assumptions for the 2006-based national population projections. *Population Trends*, 131: 19–27.

Johnson, M. (2006) Refugees and other new migrants: a review of the evidence on successful approaches to integration. London: Home Office.

Jolly, M., Sebire, N., Harris, J., Robinson, S. and Regan, L. (2000) The risks associated with pregnancy in women aged 35 years or older. *Human Reproduction*, 15(11): 2433–2437.

Jones, C.C.G., Jomeen, J., Haymer, M., *et al.* (2014) The impact of peer support in the context of perinatal mental illness: a meta-ethnography. *Midwifery*, 30: 491–498.

Jones, R.E. and Lopez, K.H. (2014) *Human Reproductive Biology*, 4th edn. Amsterdam: Elsevier.

Keeling, J. and Birch, L. (2004) Asking pregnant women about domestic abuse. *British Journal of Midwifery*, 12(12): 746–749.

Kenyon, A.P. (2010) Effect of age on maternal and fetal outcomes. *British Journal of Midwifery*, 18(6): 358–362.

Kesmodel, U., Wisborg, K., Olsen, S.F., Henriksen, T.B. and Secher, N.J. (2002) Moderate alcohol intake in pregnancy and the risk of spontaneous abortion. *Alcohol and Alcoholism*, 37(1): 87–92.

Klee, H., Jackson, M. and Lewis, S. (2002) *Drug Misuse and Motherhood*. London: Routledge.

Knight, M., Kenyon, S., Brocklehurst, P., *et al.* (eds) (2014) on behalf of MBRRACEUK. *Saving Lives, Improving Mothers' Care – Lessons Learned to Inform Future Maternity Care from the UK and Ireland. Confidential Enquiries into Maternal Deaths and Morbidity 2009–12*. Oxford: National Perinatal Epidemiology Unit.

Künzle, R., Mueller, M.D., Hänggi, W., Birkhäuser, M.H., Drescher, H. and Bersinger, N.A. (2002) Semen quality of male smokers and nonsmokers in infertile couples. *Fertility and Sterility*, 79(2): 287–291.

Lancaster, C., Gold, K., Flynn, H.A., *et al.* (2010) Risk factors for depressive symptoms during pregnancy: a systematic review. *American Journal of Obstetric Gynecology*, 202(1): 5–14.

Laverack, G. (2005) *Public Health: Power, Empowerment and Professional Practice*. Hampshire: Palgrave Macmillan.

Lazaro, N. (2013) *Sexually Transmitted Infections in Primary Care*, 2nd edn. London: RCGP and BASHH.

Lewis, G. (ed) (2011) Saving mothers' lives: reviewing maternal deaths to make motherhood safer 2006–2008. The eighth report of the confidential enquiries into maternal deaths in the United Kingdom. *British Journal of Obstetrics and Gynaecology*, 118 (Supplement 1).

Lindquist, A., Knight, M., Kurinczuket, J.J., *et al.* (2013) Variation in severe maternal morbidity according to socioeconomic position: a UK national case-control study. *BMJ Open*, 3(6).

Lindquist, A., Kurinczuk, J.J., Redshaw, M. and Knight, M. (2014) Experiences, utilisation and outcomes of maternity care in England among women from different socio-economic groups: findings from the 2010 National Maternity Survey. *British Journal of Obstetrics and Gynaecology*, DOI:10.1111/1471-0528.13059.

Lok, A., Vasudevan, C. and Johnson, K. (2011) *Ketamine Use in Pregnancy: Potential Life Long Effects on the Unborn Fetus [Poster]*. The Leeds Neonatal Service, www.addictionssa.org/2011/JohnsonK%20 Ketamine%20Poster.pdf, accessed 21 February 2015.

Lumley, J., Chamberlain, C., Dowswell, T., Oliver, S., Oakley, L. and Watson, L. (2009) *Interventions for Promoting Smoking Cessation During Pregnancy (Review). The Cochrane Collaboration*. Oxford: Wiley.

MacKenzie Bryers, H. and van Teijlingen, E. (2010) Risk, theory, social and medical models: a critical analysis of the concept of risk in maternity care. *Midwifery*, 26(5): 488–496.

Maggard, M.A., Yermilov, I., Li, Z., Maglione, M., Newberry, S., Suttorp, M. and Shekelle, P.G. (2008) Pregnancy and fertility following bariatric surgery: a systematic review. *JAMA*, 300(19): 2286–2296.

Manning, V. (2011) *Estimates of the Numbers of Infants (Under the Age of One Year) Living With Substance Misusing Parents*. London: NSPCC.

Marmot, M. (2010) *Fair Society, Healthy Lives (The Marmot Review)*. London: Health Observatory, www.instituteofhealthequity.org/projects/fair-society-healthy-lives-the-marmot-review, accessed 20 February 2015.

Marshall, N.E., Guild, C., Cheng, Y.W., Caughey, A.B. and Halloran, D.R. (2012) Maternal superobesity and perinatal outcomes. *American Journal of Obstetrics and Gynecology*, 206(5): 417.e1–417.e6.

Mathieu, J. (2009) What is pregorexia? *Journal of the American Dietetic Association*, 109(6): 976–979.

McBride, A. and Petersen, T. (eds) (2002) *Working with Substance Misusers: A Guide to Theory and Practice*. London: Routledge.

McDermott, E., Graham, H. and Hamilton, V. (2004) *Experiences of Being a Teenage Mother in the UK: A Report of a Systematic Review of Qualitative Studies*. London: Social and Public Health Sciences Unit.

McManus, S., Meltzer, H., Smith, J., *et al.* (2009) *Adult Psychiatric Morbidity in England, 2007: Results of a Household Survey*. London: NHS Information Centre.

Mercer, C.H., Tanton, C., Prah, P., *et al.* (2013) Changes in sexual attitudes and lifestyles in Britain through the life course and over time: findings from the National Surveys of Sexual Attitudes and Lifestyles (Natsal 3). *The Lancet* 382: 1781–1794.

Micali, N. (2008) Eating disorders and pregnancy. *Psychiatry*, 7(4): 191–193.

Micali, N., Treasure, J. and Simonoff, E. (2007) Eating disorders symptoms in pregnancy: a longitudinal study of women with recent and past eating disorders and obesity. *Journal of Psychosomatic Research*, 63(3): 297–303.

Midwifery 2020 (2010a) *Core Role of the Midwife Workstream: Final Report*. London: Midwifery 2020.

Midwifery 2020 (2010b) *Delivering Expectations*, http://midwifery2020.org.uk/documents/M2020 Deliveringexpectations-FullReport2.pdf, accessed 21 February 2015.

Mohllajee, A.P., Curtis, K.M., Morrow, B., *et al.* (2007) Pregnancy intention and its relationship to birth and maternal outcomes. *Obstetrics and Gynecology*, 109(3): 678–686.

Moss, B. (2012) *Communication Skills in Health and Social Care*, 2nd edn. London: SAGE.

Murray, L. and Andrews, L. (2005) *The Social Baby*. London: CP Publishing.

National Collaborating Centre for Mental Health (2011) *Induced Abortion and Mental Health: A Systematic Review of the Mental Health Outcomes of Induced Abortion, Including Their Prevalence and Associated Factors*. London: National Collaborating Centre for Mental Health.

National Institute for Health and Care Excellence [NICE] (2004) *Eating Disorders: Core Interventions in the Treatment and Management of Anorexia Nervosa, Bulimia Nervosa and Related Eating Disorders (NICE Guideline)*, www.nice.org.uk/guidance/cg9, accessed 20 February 2015.

National Institute for Health and Care Excellence [NICE] (2005) *Long Acting Reversible Contraception* [LARC], www.nice.org.uk/guidance/cg30, accessed 20 February 2015.

National Institute for Health and Care Excellence [NICE] (2006a) *Obesity: Guidance on the Prevention, Identification, Assessment and Management of Overweight and Obesity in Adults and Children (NICE Guideline)*, www.nice.org.uk/guidance/cg43, accessed 20 February 2015.

National Institute for Health and Care Excellence [NICE] (2006b) *Postnatal Care: Routine Postnatal Care of Women and Their Babies*, www.nice.org.uk/guidance/cg37, accessed 20 February 2015.

National Institute for Health and Care Excellence [NICE] (2008) *Antenatal Care.* www.nice.org.uk/guidance/cg62, accessed 20 February 2015.

National Institute for Health and Care Excellence [NICE] (2010a) *Pregnancy and Complex Social Factors*, www.nice.org.uk/guidance/cg110, accessed 20 February 2015.

National Institute for Health and Care Excellence [NICE] (2010b) *Quitting Smoking in Pregnancy and Following Childbirth*, www.nice.org.uk/guidance/ph26, accessed 20 February 2015.

National Institute for Health and Care Excellence [NICE] (2010c) *Weight Management Before, During and After Pregnancy*, www.nice.org.uk/guidance/ph27, accessed 20 February 2015.

National Institute for Health and Care Excellence [NICE] (2011) *Common Mental Health Disorders.* London: NICE.

National Institute for Health and Care Excellence [NICE] (2013a) *Fertility: Assessment and Treatment for People with Fertility Problems.* www.nice.org.uk/guidance/cg156, accessed 20 February 2015.

National Institute for Health and Care Excellence [NICE] (2013b) *Smoking Cessation in Secondary Care: Acute, Maternity and Mental Health Services.* London: NICE.

National Institute for Health and Care Excellence [NICE] (2014a) *Intrapartum Care.* www.nice.org.uk/guidance/cg190, accessed 20 February 2015.

National Institute for Health and Care Excellence [NICE] (2014b) *Postnatal Care.* www.nice.org.uk/guidance/cg37, accessed 20 February 2015.

National Institute for Health and Care Excellence [NICE] (2014c) *Antenatal and Postnatal Mental Health: Clinical Management and Service Guidance.* London: NICE.

National Organisation for Foetal Alcohol Syndrome [NOFAS] (2011) *Alcohol and Pregnancy: Information for Midwives.* London: NOFAS-UK.

NHS Cervical Screening Programme (NHSCSP) (2010) *Colposcopy and Programme Management Guidelines for the NHS Cervical Screening Programme*, 2nd edn. Sheffield: NHSCSP.

NHS Choices (2013a) *Causes of Down's Syndrome*, www.nhs.uk/Conditions/Downs-syndrome/Pages/Causes.aspx, accessed 20 February 2015.

NHS Choices (2013b) *Chorionic Villus Sampling: Complications*, www.nhs.uk/Conditions/Chorionic-Villus-sampling/Pages/Risks.aspx, accessed 20 February 2015.

NHS Information Centre, Lifestyles Statistics (2012) *Statistics on Obesity, Physical Activity and Diet: England.* London: NHS.

Ní Bhrolcháin, M. and Beaujouan, E. (2012) Fertility postponement is largely due to rising educational enrolment. *Population Studies: A Journal of Demography*, 66(3): 311–327.

Nottingham Clinical Trials Unit (2013) *The 35/39 Trial*, www.35-39trial.org, accessed 20 February 2015.

Nursing and Midwifery Council [NMC] (2009) *Standards for Pre-Registration Midwifery Education.* London: NMC.

Nursing and Midwifery Council [NMC] (2012) *Midwives Rules and Standards.* London: NMC.

Nursing and Midwifery Council [NMC] (2015) *The Code: Professional Standards of Practice and Behaviour for Nurses and Midwives.* London: NMC.

Nybo Andersen, A.M., Wohlfahrt, J. and Christens, P. (2000) Higher maternal age was associated with increased risks for fetal death and ectopic pregnancy. *British Medical Journal*, 320: 1707–1712.

O'Connell, M. and Duaso, M. (2014) Barriers and facilitators of midwives' use of the carbon monoxide breath test for smoking cessation in practice: a qualitative study. *MIDIRS Midwifery Digest*, 24(4): 453–458.

Office for National Statistics [ONS] (2014) *Drug Misuse: Findings from the 2013/14 Crime Survey for England and Wales London, Home Office*. www.gov.uk/government/publications/drug-misuse-findings-from-the-2013-to-2014-csew/drug-misuse-findings-for-the-201314-crime-survey-for-england-and-wales, accessed 20 February 2015.

Orbach, S. and Rubin, H. (2014) *Two for the Price of One: The Impact of Body Image During Pregnancy and After Birth*. London: Government Equalities Office.

Paananen, R., Ristikari, T., Merikukka, M., *et al.* (2013) Social determinants of mental health: a Finnish nationwide follow-up study on mental disorders. *Journal of Epidemiology and Community Health*, 67(12): 1025–1031.

Page, L. (2011) The joy of the late life baby. *Essentially MIDIRS*, 2(8): 17–21.

Painter, C. and Adams, J. (2004) *Explore, Dream Discover: Working with Holistic Models of Sexual Health and Sexuality, Self Esteem and Mental Health*. Sheffield: Centre for HIV and Sexual Health.

Passmore, H. and Chenery-Morris, S. (2013) New beginnings: factors affecting health and well-being in the neonate. In Taylor, J., Bond, E. and Woods, M. (eds) *Early Childhood Studies: A Multidisciplinary and Holistic Introduction*, 3rd edn. London: Hodder Education.

Peters, H., Byrne, L. and Tookey, P.A. (2014) Variation in mode of delivery for Public Health England (PHE). *Health Protection Report* 8, www.gov.uk/government/uploads/system/uploads/attachment_data/file/345181/Volume_8_number_24_hpr2414_AA_stis.pdf, accessed 20 February 2015.

Prentice, S. (2010) Substance misuse in pregnancy. *Obstetrics, Gynaecology and Reproductive Medicine*, 20(9): 278–283.

Price, S. (ed) (2007) *Mental Health in Pregnancy and Childbirth*. Edinburgh: Elsevier.

Prochaska, J. (1992) What causes people to change from unhealthy to healthy enhancing behaviour? In Heller, T., Bailey, L. and Patison, S. (eds) *Preventing Cancers*. Buckingham: Open University Press.

Prochaska, J. and DiClemente, C. (1983) Stages and processes of self-change of smoking: toward an integrative model of change. *Journal of Consulting and Clinical Psychology*, 51(3): 390–395.

Prochaska, J.O. and DiClemente, C.C. (1986) Toward a comprehensive model of change. In Miller, W.R. and Heather, N. (eds) *Treating Addictive Behaviours: Process of Change*. New York: Plenum Press.

Prochaska. J. and Velicer, W. (1997) The transtheoretical model of health behavior change. *American Journal of Health Promotion*, 12(1): 38–48.

Public Health England [PHE] (2013a) *PHE Alcohol Learning Resources: Fast Alcohol Screening Test [FAST]*, www.alcohollearningcentre.org.uk/Topics/Browse/BriefAdvice/?parent=4444&child=4570, accessed 20 February 2015.

Public Health England [PHE] (2013b) *PHE Alcohol Learning Resources: FRAMES*, www.alcohollearning centre.org.uk/alcoholeLearning/learning/IBA/Module4_v2/D/ALC_Session/300/tab_909.html, accessed 20 February 2015.

Public Health England [PHE] (2014) *Health Protection Report* 8(24), www.gov.uk/government/uploads/system/uploads/attachment_data/file/345181/Volume_8_number_24_hpr2414_AA_stis.pdf, accessed 1 March 2015.

Public Health England [PHE] (no date) *NHS Cervical Screening Programme*, www.cancerscreening.nhs.uk/cervical/about-cervical-screening.html, accessed 21 February 2015.

Quilliam, S. (2010) Sex during pregnancy: Yes, Yes, Yes! *Journal of Family Planning Reproductive Health Care*, 36(2): 97–98.

Rajasingam, D. and Swamy, S. (2010) Ultrasonography and the obese woman. In Richens, Y. and Lavender, T. (eds) *Care for Pregnant Women Who Are Obese.* London: Quay Books.

Raynor, M. and England, C. (2010) *Psychology for Midwives: Pregnancy, Childbirth and Puerperium.* Maidenhead: Open University Press.

RCP (2008) *Perinatal Maternal Mental Health Services.* London: Royal College of Psychiatrists.

Redshaw, R., Rowe, C., Hockley, C., *et al.* (2007) *Recorded Delivery: A National Survey of Women's Experience of Maternity Care 2006.* Oxford: National Perinatal Epidemiology Unit.

Reece, E.A., Leguizamon, G. and Wiznitzer, A. (2009) Gestational diabetes: the need for a common ground. *Lancet* 373(9677): 1789–1797.

Richens, Y. and Fiennes, A. (2010) Bariatic surgery and care of the pregnant women. In Richens, Y. and Lavender, T. (eds) *Care for Pregnant Women Who Are Obese* (pp19–27). London: Quay Books.

Richens, Y. and Lavender, T. (eds) (2010) *Care for Pregnant Women Who Are Obese.* London: Quay Books.

Rilling, J.K. (2013) The neural and hormonal bases of human parental care. *Neuropsychologia*, 51(4): 731–747.

Robinson, J. (1996) The SEX model of sexual health. *British Journal of Midwifery*, 4(8): 420–424.

Rogers, R., Deven, N. and Wan, G. (2012) *Body Gossip.* London: Rickshaw Publishing.

Rollans, M., Schmied, V., Austin, M., *et al.* (2013) 'We just ask some questions …': the process of antenatal psychosocial assessment by midwives. *Midwifery*, 29(8): 935–942.

Roos, N., Sahlin, L., Ekman-Ordeberg, G., Kieler, H. and Stephansson, O. (2010) Maternal risk factors for postterm pregnancy and Cesarean delivery following labor induction. *Acta Obstetricia et Gynecologica Scandinavica*, 89(8): 1003–1010.

Royal College of Midwives (1999) *Domestic Abuse in Pregnancy.* London: RCM.

Royal College of Midwives (2012) *Evidence-Based Guidelines for Midwifery-Led Care in Labour: Good Practice Points*, 5th edn, www.rcm.org.uk/sites/default/files/Introduction.pdf, accessed 20 February 2015.

Royal College of Obstetricians and Gynaecologists [ROCG] (1997) *Violence Against Women.* London: RCOG Press.

Royal College of Obstetricians and Gynaecologists [RCOG] Faculty of Sexual and Reproductive Healthcare (2009a) *UK Medical Eligibility Criteria for Contraceptive Use.* London: RCOG.

Royal College of Obstetricians and Gynaecologists [RCOG] (2009b) *RCOG Statement on Later Maternal Age*, www.rcog.org.uk/what-we-do/campaigning-and-opinions/statement/rcog-statement-later-maternal-age, accessed 21 February 2015.

Royal College of Obstetricians and Gynaecologists [RCOG] (2011) *Management of Women with Mental Health Issues During Pregnancy and the Postnatal Period.* London: RCOG.

Royal College of Psychiatrists (2002) *Domestic Violence.* CR102. London: RCP.

Royal College of Psychiatrists (2008) *Perinatal Maternal Mental Health Services.* London: RCP.

Royal College of Psychiatrists (2014) *Eating Disorders: Key Facts*, www.rcpsych.ac.uk/healthadvice/problemsdisorders/eatingdisorderskeyfacts.aspx, accessed 21 February 2015.

Sasieni, P., Adams, J. and Cuzick, J. (2003) Benefit of cervical screening at different ages: evidence from the UK audit of screening histories. *British Journal of Cancer*, 89: 88–93.

Schytt, E. and Waldenström, U. (2013) How well does midwifery education prepare for clinical practice? Exploring the views of Swedish students, midwives and obstetricians. *Midwifery*, 29(2): 102–109.

Scriven, A. (2010) *Promoting Health: A Practical Guide: Forewords: Linda Ewles and Ina Simnett; Richard Parish*. Edinburgh: Baillière Tindall.

SIGN (2012) *Management of Perinatal Mood Disorders*. Edinburgh: SIGN.

Sinclair, M. and Stockdale, J. (2011) Achieving optimal birth using salutogenesis in routine antenatal education. *Evidence Based Midwifery*, 9(3): 75.

Siney, C. (ed) (1999) *Pregnancy and Drug Misuse*, 2nd edn. Hale: Books for Midwives Press.

Smith, C.G., Pell, J.P. and Dobbie, R. (2003) Interpregnancy interval and risk of preterm birth and neonatal death: retrospective cohort study. *BMJ*, 327: 851.

Smith, K., Coleman, K., Eder, S. and Hall, P. (2011) *Homicides, Firearm Offences and Intimate Violence 2009/10*. Supplementary Volume 2 to *Crime in England and Wales*. London: Home Office (Crown Copyright).

Social Exclusion Unit (SEU) (1999) *Teenage Pregnancy*. London: The Stationery Office, http://dera.ioe.ac.uk/15086/1/teenage-pregnancy.pdf, accessed 20 February 2015.

Society of Sexual Health Advisors [SSHA] (2004) *The Manual for Sexual Health Advisors*. London: SSHA.

Sonnenberg, P., Clifton, S., Beddows, S., *et al.* (2013) Prevalence, risk factors, and uptake of interventions for sexually transmitted infections in Britain: findings from the National Surveys of Sexual Attitudes and Lifestyles (Natsal 3). *The Lancet*, 382: 1795–1806.

Stables, D. and Rankin, J. (2010) *Physiology in Childbearing: With Anatomy and Related Biosciences*, 3rd edn. Edinburgh: Baillière Tindall Elsevier.

Stapleton, H. (2010) *Surviving Teenage Motherhood: Myths and Realities*. Basingstoke: Palgrave Macmillan.

Steel, N., Blakeborough, L. and Nicholas, S. (2011) *Supporting High-Risk Victims of Domestic Violence: A Review of Multi-Agency Risk Assessment Conferences (MARACs)*, www.gov.uk/government/uploads/system/uploads/attachment_data/file/116536/horr55-summary.pdf, accessed 20 February 2015.

Stein, Z. and Susser, M. (2000) The risks of having children in later life: social advantage may make up for biological disadvantage. *British Medical Journal*, 320(7521): 1681–1682.

Stice, E. (2002) Risk and maintenance factors for eating pathology: a metaanalytic review. *Psychological Bulletin*, 128: 825–848.

Sullivan, R., Perry, R., Mendoza, R., *et al.* (2011) Infant bonding and attachment to the caregiver: insights from basic and clinical science. *Clinics in Perinatology*, 38(4): 643–655.

Sutcliffe, A.G., Barnes, J., Belsky, J., Gardiner, J. and Melhuish, E. (2012) The health and development of children born to older mothers in the United Kingdom: observational study using longitudinal cohort data. *BMJ*, 345(e5116), www.bmj.com/content/345/bmj.e5116.full?ijkey=2dAjhG7v8Zfv5Qw&keytype=ref

Sutherland, G., Brown, S., Yelland, J., *et al.* (2013) Applying a social disparities lens to obesity in pregnancy to inform efforts to intervene. *Midwifery*, 29(4): 338–343.

Swann, C., Bowe, K., McCormick, G. and Kosmin, M. (2003) *Teenage Pregnancy and Parenthood: A Review of Reviews*. London: Health Development Agency.

te Velde, E. and Pearson, E.P. (2002) The variability of female reproductive ageing. *Human Reproduction, Update*, 8: 141–154.

Thyrian, J.R., Freyer-Adam, J., Hannover, W., *et al.* (2010) Population-based smoking cessation in women post partum: adherence to motivational interviewing in relation to client characteristics and behavioural outcomes. *Midwifery*, 26(2): 202–210.

Townsend, C.L., Byrne, L., Cortina-Borja, M., *et al.* (2014) Earlier initiation of ART and further decline in mother-to-child HIV transmission rates, 2000–2011. *AIDS*, 28(7): 1049–1057.

Treacy, A., Robson, M. and O'Herlihy, C. (2006) Dystocia increases with advancing maternal age. *American Journal of Obstetrics and Gynecology*, 195(3): 760–763.

Treasure, J. (2012) Eating disorders. *Medicine*, 40(11): 607–612.

Trevithick, P. (2010) *Social Work Skills: A Practice Handbook*, 2nd edn. Maidenhead: Open University.

Trussell, J. and Portman, D. (2013) The creeping pearl: why has the rate of contraceptive failure increased in clinical trials of combined hormonal contraceptive pills? *Contraception*, 88: 604–610.

von Brummen, H.J., Bruinse, H.W., van de Pol, G., Heintz, A.P.M. and van der Vaart, C.H. (2006) Which factors determine the sexual function 1 year after childbirth? *British Journal of Obstetrics and Gynaecology*, 113: 914–918.

Walby, S. and Allen, J. (2004) *Domestic Violence, Sexual Assault and Stalking: Findings from the British Crime Survey*. London: Home Office.

Walsh, J., Mahony, R., Armstrong, F., *et al.* (2011) Ethnic variation between white European women in labour outcomes in a setting in which the management of labour is standardised – a healthy migrant effect? *BJOG: An International Journal of Obstetrics and Gynaecology*, 118(6): 713–718.

Wellings, K. and Kane, R. (1999) Trends in teenage pregnancy in England and Wales: how can we explain them? *Journal of the Royal Society of Medicine*, 92(6): 277–282.

Wellings, K., Jones, K.G., Mercer, C.H., *et al.* (2013) The prevalence of unplanned pregnancy and associated factors in Britain: findings from the third National Survey of Sexual Attitudes and Lifestyles (Natsal 3) *The Lancet*, 382: 1807–1816.

Whittaker, A. (2003) *Substance Misuse in Pregnancy: A Resource Pack for Professionals in Lothian*. Edinburgh: NHS Lothian.

Whooley, M.A., Avins, A.L., Miranda, J., *et al.* (1997) Case-finding instruments for depression: two questions are as good as many. *Journal of General Internal Medicine*, 12: 439–445.

Williams, A.A. and Wright, K.S. (2014) Engaging families through motivational interviewing. *Pediatric Clinics of North America*, 61(5): 907–921.

Wilson, A. (2010) Craving to quit. *Midwives*, March, p50.

Women's Aid (2015) *Survivor's Handbook: Making a Safety Plan*, www.womensaid.org.uk/domestic-violence-survivors- handbook.asp?section=000100010008000100310005, accessed 20 February 2015.

World Health Organization (1946) *Preamble to the Constitution of the World Health Organization as Adopted by the International Health Conference, New York, 19–22 June, 1946*; signed on 22 July 1946 by the representatives of 61 States (Official Records of the World Health Organization, no. 2, p100) and entered into force on 7 April 1948.

World Health Organization (2006) *Defining Sexual Health.* Report of a technical consultation on sexual health, 28–31 January. Geneva: WHO.

Yangmei, L., Townend, J., Rowe, R., Knight, M., Brocklehurst, P. and Hollowell, J. (2014) The effect of maternal age and planned place of birth on intrapartum outcomes in healthy women with straightforward pregnancies: secondary analysis of the Birthplace National Prospective Cohort Study. *British Medical Journal,* 4, BMJ Open 2014;4:e004026 doi:10.1136/bmjopen-2013-004026.

Zumpe, J., Dormon, O., Jefferies, J., *et al.* (2012) *Childbearing Among UK Born and Non-UK Born Women Living in the UK.* London: Office for National Statistics.

Index